More Praise for *100 Questions & Answers About Brain Tumors,*
Second Edition

"Dr. Stark-Vance and M.L. Dubay's book has been an absolutely marvelous and invaluable resource for my patients and their families as they try to grasp the realities of dealing with a malignant brain tumor."

Richard L. Weiner, MD, FACS

"*100 Questions & Answers About Brain Tumors, Second Edition,* is a valuable resource for newly diagnosed brain tumor patients and caregivers who have many questions and are in need of answers. Dr. Stark-Vance and M.L. Dubay form the perfect team in presenting the issues from the medical and the patient's perspectives. This book is at the top of my recommended reading list."

Jerry D. Kline
Brain Tumor Survivor

"Dr. Stark-Vance and M.L. Dubay offer a complete guide to the information survivors need to confront their 'beast' during this very uncertain, difficult, and challenging journey. This second publication is packed with powerful information to lead brain tumor survivors with empowerment and strength."

Sheryl R. Shetsky
umor Survivor
or Association
www.fbta.info

"This book provides an _____ ___, user-friendly resource for brain tumor patients and their loved ones. Fortunately there are a growing number of medications and treatment strategies that are making a difference and helping patients every day. Unavoidably, the downside of this growth is an increase in the complexity of information and options out there for brain tumor patients. Dr. Stark-Vance, an outstanding and dedicated clinician, has put together a terrific overview to help patients and their loved ones get on track and stay there in their fight against this disease."

David A. Reardon, MD
Associate Deputy Director,
The Preston Robert Tisch Brain Tumor Center
Associate Professor, Department of Surgery
Associate Professor, Department of Pediatrics
Durham, North Carolina

"I wish that I could've had a book like this when I was first diagnosed with a brain tumor. Dr. Stark-Vance and M.L. Dubay bring invaluable dual perspectives to a complex, challenging medical situation. Their comprehensive information and affirmation will educate both patients and caregivers."

Heather Foster Hall
Nine-Year Brain Tumor Survivor
(pictured on the cover of this book)

"*100 Questions & Answers About Brain Tumors, Second Edition,* is a must-have resource for our brain tumor patients, whether they are newly diagnosed or just needing some clarification or reassurance. The book is easy to read and is pertinent to the questions our patients and their caregivers ask."

Sandi McDermott, RN, MSN, NEA-BC
Manager Neurosciences, Medical City Dallas Hospital
Dallas, Texas

100 Questions & Answers About Brain Tumors
Second Edition

Virginia Stark-Vance, MD

M.L. Dubay

JONES AND BARTLETT PUBLISHERS
Sudbury, Massachusetts
BOSTON   TORONTO   LONDON   SINGAPORE

blishers   Jones and Bartlett Publishers
                    International
y   Barb House, Barb Mews
       L5V 1J2   London W6 7PA
                    United Kingdom

ugh most bookstores and online booksellers. To contact Jones and Bartlett Publishers directly, call 800-832-0034, fax 978-443-8000, or visit our website, www.jbpub.com.

Substantial discounts on bulk quantities of Jones and Bartlett's publications are available to corporations, professional associations, and other qualified organizations. For details and specific discount information, contact the special sales department at Jones and Bartlett via the above contact information or send an email to specialsales@jbpub.com

The authors, editor, and publisher have made every effort to provide accurate information. However, they are not responsible for errors, omissions, or for any outcomes related to the use of the contents of this book and take no responsibility for the use of the products and procedures described. Treatments and side effects described in this book may not be applicable to all people; likewise, some people may require a dose or experience a side effect that is not described herein. Drugs and medical devices are discussed that may have limited availability controlled by the Food and Drug Administration (FDA) for use only in a research study or clinical trial. Research, clinical practice, and government regulations often change the accepted standard in this field. When consideration is being given to use of any drug in the clinical setting, the healthcare provider or reader is responsible for determining FDA status of the drug, reading the package insert, and reviewing prescribing information for the most up-to-date recommendations on dose, precautions, and contraindications, and determining the appropriate usage for the product. This is especially important in the case of drugs that are new or seldom used.

Production Credits
Executive Publisher: Chris Davis
Editorial Assistant: Sara Cameron
Production Director: Amy Rose
Associate Production Editor: Jessica deMartin
Manufacturing and Inventory Control
    Supervisor: Amy Bacus
Composition: Glyph International
Printing and Binding: Malloy, Inc.

Cover Credits
Cover Design: Carolyn Downer
Cover Printing: Malloy, Inc.
Cover Image: © Jeanette Gorsky

Library of Congress Cataloging-in-Publication Data
Stark-Vance, Virginia.
    100 questions & answers about brain tumors / Virginia Stark-Vance, M.L. Dubay.—2nd ed.
    p. cm.
    Includes index.
    ISBN-13: 978-0-7637-6054-0
    ISBN-10: 0-7637-6054-4
    1. Brain—Tumors--Miscsellanea. 2. Brain—Tumors—Popular works. I. Dubay, M.L.
(Mary Louise) II. Title. III. Title: 100 question and answers about brain tumors. IV. Title:
One hundred question and answers about brain tumors.
    RC280.B7S79 2011
    616.99'481—dc22   2009041093

6048

Printed in the United States of America
13 12 11 10   10 9 8 7 6 5 4 3 2 1

In 2000, Heather Foster Hall (who was also on the cover of the first edition of this book) was a busy working mother of two young children (ages 1 and 3) when she developed unusual headaches, leading to the diagnosis of anaplastic astrocytoma. Her diagnosis was especially agonizing to her family, as Heather's father had succumbed to anaplastic astrocytoma nearly three decades earlier, when Heather was a young child. Because her tumors could not be surgically removed, Heather was treated with radiation therapy and Temodar. Nine years later, Heather remains in complete remission, and she credits God and the wisdom of her doctors with her recovery.

"All I wanted was more time . . . time to watch my babies grow up and to see their personalities and little souls develop. Every day that I wake up and get to be part of their lives is a blessing."

Heather was photographed by Jeanette Gorsky, the wife of artist Vladimir Gorsky, who died of glioblastoma in 2008.

Contents

Contents

Every year, more than 190,000 Americans experience the shock, fear, and confusion inherent with the words, "You have a brain tumor." If you are reading this book, you or someone close to you has most likely been impacted in some way by this most devastating diagnosis.

The good news is that medical and scientific researchers have made considerable progress in our knowledge and understanding of brain tumors. For example, today we know much more than we did even 5 years ago about genetic and cellular alterations that may cause brain tumors. We are also better at meeting the special needs of brain tumor patients. An increasing number of research centers across the country have established neuroscience departments, which include specialized programs for brain tumor patients, and there have been some significant breakthroughs in imaging techniques that are aiding brain tumor diagnostics and ensuring more precise brain tumor surgery. Clinical trials throughout the United States are investigating a wide variety of new therapies, including brain tumor vaccines and targeted compounds. There has been an explosion of interest in brain tumors, and a greater commitment to the patients and families living with this devastating disease. As a result, there are more patient education programs and support groups, and walks and events to support brain tumor research, than ever before.

The late Senator Ted Kennedy's diagnosis brought national attention to the reality of brain tumors, a disease that affects all ages, genders, races, and socioeconomic levels. And yet there is much we do not know in terms of why some people develop brain tumors and others do not. We know that brain tumors are the number one cause of solid tumor death in children, and that both men and women can receive a brain tumor diagnosis although women are more likely to have a brain tumor that is benign. Some research has shown that brain tumors are more common in certain geographic areas and professions, but the reasons are unclear.

The American Brain Tumor Association (ABTA) has been a strong advocate for brain tumor research and patient education. Millions of dollars are raised through volunteer events to fund ABTA research grants, develop educational materials for patients and caregivers, and host regional meetings to present the latest brain tumor research. It is our goal to continue to help brain tumor patients find accurate sources of information that can help them make informed decisions about their treatment and care. For those individuals living with a brain tumor, as well as their loved ones and caregivers, *100 Questions & Answers About Brain Tumors, Second Edition,* is a valuable guide for navigating the complex and often frightening brain tumor journey. Its logical format and conversational tone make it an ideal introduction to the diagnostic tests and treatment decisions that the new patient must face.

This second edition expands on the original book with more illustrations, up-to-date discussions of the latest treatments, and more resources for the caregiver. Author Virginia Stark-Vance is a practicing physician with extensive experience in research and clinical trials who writes with clarity and precision. Her co-author and patient, M.L. Dubay, is a 9-year brain tumor survivor who has experienced the terror of diagnosis, the anxiety of dozens of magnetic resonance imaging (MRI) scans, and the shared joy of hundreds of brain tumor survivors through her work with volunteer organizations. These women obviously share a common interest in educating and encouraging brain tumor patients and their caregivers.

100 Questions & Answers About Brain Tumors, Second Edition is an important companion for brain tumor patients, family members, and caregivers, as well as physicians and other health care professionals caring for individuals living with this disease.

Elizabeth M. Wilson
Executive Director,
American Brain Tumor Association

The first edition of this book by Dr. Virginia Stark-Vance and Mary Louise ("M.L.") Dubay fulfilled a great need, as will this newly updated version.

As the authors acknowledge in their introduction to this second edition: "Fortunately, shortly after the first edition of *100 Questions & Answers About Brain Tumors* was published, there were new treatments, new procedures, and new diagnostic tests that became available for brain tumor patients."

With brain tumors, we all hope that significant progress will continuously be made and that what we know today in terms of treatment will be rapidly augmented by promising new therapies tomorrow. That is the "fortunate" thing, and the aim of most who are diagnosed with a brain tumor, particularly a malignant primary brain tumor, is to be one of the people who will benefit from major new advances on the road to a cure for this devastating disease.

We in the International Brain Tumour Alliance are in contact with brain tumor patients and caregivers all over the world. Often we hear from them that, on diagnosis, they feel as though they have suddenly become unwilling travelers in a strange and surreal landscape. They don't speak or understand the complicated medical language, and they don't know how to get from A to B in terms of navigating support and benefit services. Most of all, however, they are filled with fear and dread of the unknown road ahead. They have no map, no compass, and no anchor.

Thus, the book that you hold in your hands is very valuable. Virginia Stark-Vance provides the professional perspective in concise, easy-to-understand layperson's language. She covers a large number of crucial topics to help patients, their families, and their caregivers find their footing on this journey. M.L. Dubay, who was diagnosed with an anaplastic oligodendroglioma in July 2000, provides the patient perspective in a way that only someone who is herself affected by this disease can—that is, with great insight and practical, first-hand experience.

When a brain tumor enters your life, your priorities completely change and you begin to live what is called "the new normal." This book will help you approach the "new normal" and learn to live it.

Every year, 200,000 people worldwide develop a primary malignant brain tumor.[1]

Brain tumors—of which there are over 120 different types— can combine the worst of the neurological diseases with the worst of cancer. Depending on the type and grade and in which part of the brain it is located, a brain tumor can affect cognition, physical abilities, personality, and emotion. Brain tumors afflict people of any age—from tiny babies to older persons—with equal ferocity, regardless of background, race, or geographic location.

Brain tumors "also threaten to steal what is held so highly as the essence of human life: the mind and the spirit."[2]

The causes of brain tumors are, as yet, largely unknown so there are neither prevention programs for them nor any realistic screening programs. There is no known preventive option by healthy living, diet, or exercise, although all of these things are important in living with a brain tumor.

Besides the patient, countless others—such as caregivers and family members—are deeply impacted by the effects of the brain tumor on their loved ones. We know this because we have been there ourselves, as caregivers to a beloved wife and a treasured son.

The challenges of day-to-day living that are often faced by a brain tumor patient are also experienced by that patient's caregiver. Thus, cancer survivorship becomes not a one-person journey through the maze of medical, social, and economic aspects of the disease but a journey that includes caregivers, family members, and friends as well.

Thus, we also recommend this book to those whose role in this journey will be to support, provide practical help, and emotionally bolster those who have been diagnosed with a brain tumor. A caregiver's role can be daunting, and very often a patient's quality of life can be affected by the way in which that caring is provided. A calm, knowledgeable caregiver is crucial, and we would very much like to see the additional needs of caregivers acknowledged by more comprehensive support and information such as that contained in this book.

We feel that this book provides many of those answers to questions that caregivers always wanted to know but might have been afraid to ask!

Great personal discipline must be exerted by all who are involved with the patient's care to preserve a sense of hope in this journey. It will ease the path, but it needs to be a realistic hope, in which delusion does not play a role—hope that does not ignore the great challenges and constraints of existing therapies.

We are all different people, as unique and individual as our own fingerprints. A brain tumor diagnosis affects people in different ways, whether we are the patient, family, or caregiver.

Although it's true that a brain tumor diagnosis imposes enormous stresses and strains on all whose lives it might touch, it has also been the catalyst for great achievements.

The devastation wreaked by brain tumors has spurred the global neuro-oncology community to develop more effective treatments. The efforts are worldwide and increasing in scope. We in the International Brain Tumour Alliance attend brain tumor conferences all over the world, and each time we do there are more and more researchers, clinicians, and allied health care professionals filling delegates' seats that only a few short years ago might have been left empty. We are seeing an unprecedented focus on more research into the causes of and treatments for brain tumors; however, there is a desperate and urgent need for even more of this work. Any brain tumor patient and his or her loved ones will tell you that advances in treatment and care can never happen quickly enough!

In addition, we are seeing the proliferation of brain tumor patient and caregiver groups, both "actual" and "virtual." These organizations and worldwide online facilities are also invaluable in providing information and support.

We take inspiration from those brain tumor patients who, for whatever as yet unknown reason, live well and live beyond their original prognoses, and we are seeing more and more of these long-term survivors. Their relative longevity gives great hope to others who travel on the same journey.

Around the world, every minute of every day, hundreds of thousands of brain tumor patients and caregivers meet the challenge of surviving their disease with courage and determination.

Virginia Stark-Vance and M.L. Dubay's second edition of *100 Questions & Answers About Brain Tumors* provides a vital road map for these challenges.

Finally, and to you whose unwanted journey with a brain tumor has led you to read this book, we wish you hope with which to confront your circumstances, with which to live each day as it comes, and with which to guide you as you travel. With the international medical, research, and patient/caregiver community all working together to develop better treatments, we do believe that one day a cure will be found.

Denis Strangman
Chair, IBTA

Kathy Oliver
Co-Director, IBTA

Notes:
1. Estimates supplied by the Central Brain Tumor Registry of the United States based on GLOBOCAN 2002.
2. Khalili, Yasmin. Ongoing transitions: the impact of a malignant brain tumour on patient and family *AXON* 2007; 28(3):5.

Fortunately, shortly after the first edition of *100 Questions & Answers About Brain Tumors* was published, there were new treatments, new procedures, and new diagnostic tests that became available for brain tumor patients. Although it can seem a bit daunting for writers to keep up with the latest information, it isn't—it's impossible. It's hard to write or update a book so that patients can have access to the latest information, but it's exciting that so much new information is available.

M.L. and I conceived this book as a guide to the newly diagnosed brain tumor patient, who may still be in the hospital recovering from surgery. We wanted to include the basic information that any patient needs to understand the terminology, the diagnostic tests, and the overview of treatment options now available. But it's becoming more apparent that, as the need for more specific information grows, the Internet has become "the next book to read." We hope that this book will serve as a guide to understanding some of the basics that will allow the patient to make the next step with confidence and not confusion.

For me, one of the very best aspects of taking care of brain tumor patients is that they all want to get well. After all, how can anything be more frightening than losing any part of the very organ that makes us human? But getting well means "a return to health," not just living through another day. We may all have different definitions as to what constitutes a quality of life, but we know what it's not. What's the first question someone usually asks when they find out they have to take chemotherapy: "What are the side effects?" Patients want to know that it's worth feeling bad for a while in the hope that the effects of the tumor will improve or at least be kept at bay.

Since I've never had a brain tumor, it would be dishonest of me to try to explain what chemotherapy, radiation, and surgery are like. However, M.L. has been there, done that, and gotten the T shirt, so to speak; and her contributions to this guide are therefore invaluable. As a 9-year survivor of a malignant glioma, M.L. has been through most of the procedures and tests described in this book, and it is her matter-of-fact description of them that give this book its heart and soul. As I mentioned in the first edition, M.L. is the kind of person you could trust to give you her honest opinion. She's intelligent, compassionate, but above all, very practical. As someone who worked in a demanding profession before, during, and after her diagnosis in 2000, she understands the struggle to keep life and work as normal as possible while juggling appointments, scans, and treatment-related fatigue. Her comments throughout the book reflect her experience not only with her own illness, but what she has learned over the last several years from fellow brain tumor survivors and recently, caring for her father while he was terminally ill. M.L. and I agreed that we wanted this edition to be more helpful to the caregiver, who, next to the patient, is the most important person on the treatment team.

Next to M.L., my family—my daughter Joy, who "volunteered" me to Jones and Bartlett to write the first edition; and my son Ted, who's kept my computer running all these years—deserve a lot of credit for their work behind the scenes. Joy, the artist and athlete of the family, keeps me abreast of the world outside the hospital (and seemed truly shocked when I told her I knew the names of the Jonas Brothers). Ted has taught me how to text, updates me on iPhone apps, and recommends downloads for my Apple TV. Ted and Joy have given me more joy than I've ever deserved, and they have often been neglected because of my clinical responsibilities. My apologies!

My other family—the office staff—keep me on schedule, but also keep me humble. They tease me about my rabbits, my messy desk, and my doctor's scrawl. My office manager, Paula, is the genius who actually makes my practice run. That woman can do anything! You couldn't ask for a better friend, and my patients quickly learn that she will move Heaven and Earth for them.

Some of my other patients and colleagues have made significant contributions to the book. In fact, my patient Dorothy and her husband Les have also made significant contributions to brain tumor treatment. In 2004, when Dorothy was still taking CPT-11, her husband read on the Internet about a new drug that had just been approved for colon cancer. He thought that this new drug, Avastin, which is the first of a new group of antiangiogenesis drugs, might be effective against Dorothy's tumor, and they suggested that we add Avastin to Dorothy's regimen. Within the first month, a substantial portion of the tumor disappeared. Shortly thereafter, Dorothy and Les told many of the other patients they knew about her success, leading to a clinical trial for my own patients. It seemed so successful that I immediately discussed the results with my friend Henry Friedman at Duke and, as they say, the rest is history. Avastin was approved by the Federal Drug Administration (FDA) in May 2009 based on its success in tumors like Dorothy's.

Other patients, including Jerry Kline, James Robinson, Doug Cooper, Don Adair, Valerie Simonds, and Steve Coffman, have written extensively about their experiences with treatment and recovery. They have helped countless newly diagnosed patients avoid some of the land mines: insurance denials, long term side effects, and dealing with recurrent disease. My patient Jeannie Murphy, who died after a 9-year battle with glioblastoma, inspired her family and friends to continue to help other brain tumor patients, especially financially. These tireless volunteers, led by Jeannie's mother Mary Lee Houghton, created the Legacy Brain Foundation in 2006 to raise money to help patients with the cost of their treatment. The Legacy Brain Foundation now reviews dozens of grant applications every year to help patients in the Dallas–Fort Worth area who are struggling with medical expenses. I wish every community could offer financial assistance to brain tumor patients, many of whom have become disabled or who have lost their insurance coverage. What a wonderful legacy that Jeannie began because of her constant desire to reach out to other patients! I feel that I've been blessed with some of the kindest, most generous patients in the world.

There are many other friends and colleagues who have contributed to the second edition. Dr. Timothy Nichols, who reviewed the chapter on radiation therapy for the first edition, offered numerous helpful comments for the second edition. Dr. Martin Lazar has been a constant source of encouragement for my treatment protocols and was pivotal in developing the new neuro-oncology unit at Medical City Dallas Hospital. Dr. Lazar also recently completed a very comprehensive, lavishly illustrated website of his own, www.dallasneurosurgery.com, which also provides neurosurgery patients with detailed care instructions. Dr. Mike Desaloms and Dr. Richard Weiner, have provided information and illustrations for the section on intra-operative MRI. Dr. Desaloms, Dr. Weiner, and the other neurosurgeons from Dallas Neurosurgical Associates have referred hundreds of patients over the last several years and have never hesitated to help out-of-town patients schedule surgery or Gamma Knife as quickly as possible. Dr. Steve Brem has been a good friend and strong supporter of my clinical studies with antiangiogenesis. Dr. Brent Alford in Fort Worth is a valued collaborator whose neurosurgery skills and gracious "bedside manner" have blessed many mutual patients. Dr. Robert Leroy is a world-class seizure expert who supplied me with a wealth of information regarding the latest in epilepsy drugs. Finally, the neuroradiologists at Southwest Diagnostic Center have had an infinite amount of patience with me as I constantly badgered them with questions about MRI scans.

There are many other doctors, nurses, and other colleagues who, on a daily basis, *care* for patients—a term that means more than writing prescriptions, starting intravenous lines, and closing incisions. They look at all aspects of a patient's life to examine what treatment is truly best for the patient. For example, I consulted on a delightful woman this week who has a very large tumor, likely a metastasis from a melanoma diagnosed years ago. I discussed her case with a very competent, but no-nonsense neurosurgeon, who agreed that she needed surgery right away. But he declined to perform the surgery, saying that she would be better served to have the tumor removed by one of his friends in Houston, since all of her adult children live there.

I was surprised and pleased that he had made his decision based on *her personal circumstances*, not on my admittedly short-sighted assessment that this Dallas resident should have her surgery in Dallas. Isn't that what we all want—what's best for the patient?

Although the advances in the diagnosis and treatment of brain tumors over the last few years have been exciting, it is still sobering to consider how many patients both in our country and worldwide do not have access to treatment. While, thanks to the Internet, patients and caregivers have more information about treatment options than ever before, that does not always translate into finding a way to *receive* treatment. Sometimes a patient wants to try a drug that is reported to be promising, but insurance will not cover it because it has not been approved for use in brain tumors. Most drugs are far too expensive for patients to pay for without insurance coverage. It is also increasingly common that physicians are refusing to give patients certain medications because insurance reimburses the physician for less than the cost of the drug! Also, since insurance reimbursement to the physician may take months, a patient may receive several doses of an expensive drug that is ultimately denied. This is particularly a problem for brain tumor patients and their doctors, since very few drugs are "approved" for use in gliomas, and for the rare tumors, *all* drugs could be considered experimental (and therefore not covered by insurance). Is it any wonder that some large cities do not even have a neuro-oncologist?

The current treatments used for brain tumors, particularly malignant gliomas, prolong life but do not necessarily cure the disease. Because of the high cost of treatment (easily $100,000+ for surgery, radiation, and several months of chemotherapy), some critics of the health care system argue that such money is better spent on vaccines and other disease-prevention strategies. Fortunately, you may say, treatment for malignant glioma patients in the United States is not denied. But what if the government cut reimbursement to neurosurgeons thirty percent? What if the National Institutes of Health's neuro-oncology budget was cut 15%? What if Medicare allowed only four brain scans a year? What if only 6 months of Temodar were reimbursed, based on the results of the original European trial? These are all possible scenarios, as Congress debates how to control spiraling health care costs.

The problem is particularly frustrating because I truly believe that we are closer than ever to understanding how cancers grow and spread in the brain, and how to disrupt their blood supply, and stop their invasion. More patients are living longer, and some are cured. But we have no idea how to identify people at risk for developing a brain tumor, and "early" diagnosis is impossible. Anyone can develop a brain tumor—even a member of Congress. And, as I found when caring for Mike Synar, the Congressman from Oklahoma who died of a glioblastoma in 1996—we desperately need more research, not less; more clinical trials, not fewer; more access to promising drugs *now*.

I look back on the years since then and I am so very grateful for the opportunities I have had to care for patients at the most challenging times of their lives. I am humbled that they trusted me enough to let me share a part of their lives. I can't begin to describe the admiration I have for them and their families. Even the patients who are demanding teach me how to see them as people God created; He cares for them, and I should follow His example. After all, I have many faults and failures of my own; and yet, I know that God loves me. If I could love my patients and their families as He does, they would be at peace, whatever the outcome.

Virginia Stark-Vance, MD

ooooo

I celebrated 9 years of being cancer free in July 2009 and it is very exhilarating to mark that date every year! I should tell you that I celebrate more frequently than just once a year . . . especially since July 2008 when I had an episode while vacationing in Charleston, South Carolina. It all happened in a flash—literally one day I was fine and the next day I was in the hospital intensive care unit (ICU) after experiencing multiple tonic-clonic seizures (formerly known as gran mal seizures). I had a tube down my throat to help me breathe and was "out of it" because the doctors had to give me a significant amount of Dilantin to stop my seizures.

My husband and family thought my brain tumor had recurred; however, after multiple MRI and CAT scans the medical staff indicated that it had not—a huge and obvious relief! The hospital released me after about 3 days and the only side effect that I experienced was that I had trouble talking and was hoarse as a result of having the tube down my throat. On the other hand, my husband and family were in shock. They couldn't believe that we all had to experience this very frightening situation less than a week after celebrating another anniversary of my being cancer-free.

This was just another reminder to me that none of us know what is going to happen from day to day. It was at that point that I decided I needed to do something different in my life, because life really is too short to not enjoy what you do every day! I continued to search my heart and I prayed a lot about what I was really supposed to be doing here on this Earth. This was the beginning of several major changes in my life since we wrote the first edition of this book 5 years ago.

At about this same time, my father's health had started to decline rapidly. He was also a cancer survivor, but was in his late seventies when he was diagnosed with his first cancer (colon). A couple of years later, he was diagnosed with his second primary cancer (bladder) and he survived that one, too. My father was a real fighter! His third primary cancer was diagnosed in late 2005 and that's the one that hit him the hardest. It was esophageal (throat) cancer and it was already at stage 4 (and my father had never smoked a cigarette, pipe, or cigar in his entire life). He came through surgery (12 hours), radiation, and chemotherapy pretty well, but his body had already been through so much. Even though he had to be tube fed, he lived for almost 3 more years. My father died on February 1, 2009 at age 81, and I was fortunate enough to be able to spend the 2 months prior to his death with him in Knoxville, Tennessee, along with my husband, mother, brothers, and sister.

The episode in Charleston made me start to think more about my future; however, the loss of my father was the first major change in my life. I had never lost anyone that close to me, and it was difficult for my entire family, but we know he is not in pain anymore and is in a better place now. The second major change was that I also decided to leave the corporate world after almost 20 years and start my own small business.

I used to make toffee every holiday season for my friends and everyone loved it. Many of them suggested that I should start my own business some day, but I was too afraid to do it. Well, after a lot of soul searching and encouragement from my husband and friends, I decided to bite the bullet and go for it! The name of the company is Toffee Treats, and as I am writing this introduction, I am also ramping up my business for what I hope is a very busy holiday season.

So, with all that said, you may be asking why Dr. Stark-Vance and I wrote this second edition. As Dr. Stark-Vance mentioned in her introduction, one of the primary reasons was due to the latest treatments that have come out since the first edition was published 5 years ago. That is not to say that the treatments that were available when I was diagnosed in 2000 are no longer effective. In fact, it is quite the contrary. The treatments that I had 9 years ago have kept me in remission, so don't feel like you must have the latest treatments in order to survive. The chemotherapy that I took 9 years ago was Temodar and it was new to the market. Today, it is still one of the best chemotherapy treatments along with radiation.

We wanted to make you aware of the advances in treatments that were not available 5 years ago. Some of these treatments, such as Avastin, have made significant impacts in the survival rate of many of Dr. Stark-Vance's patients. In fact, she was instrumental in bringing Avastin to the brain tumor community and subsequent approval by the FDA earlier this year.

This is just another example of Dr. Stark-Vance's commitment and dedication to every one of her patients. She will move mountains to make sure that each one of them has the very best treatment available for their specific tumor. I'm sure you've heard the phrase "they broke the mold when she was born," and I believe that is what they did after Dr. Stark-Vance was born. She is one of a kind!

Also, in the second edition we wanted to provide more information for caregivers of brain tumor patients. Unfortunately, caregivers don't always get the information and support they need and next to the brain cancer patient, they play one of the most important roles in the health care team.

I had my own personal experience as a caregiver for my father, earlier this year while he was on home-hospice care the last 2 months of his life. My mother had been his primary caregiver for almost 3 years as his health continued to decline. My brothers and sister were able to relieve her many times; however, there is typically only one primary caregiver and that was my mother.

During those 3 years, it was difficult for me to not be able to relieve my mother, but in December 2008, I had the opportunity to do just that. It was my turn to be the caregiver and give my siblings and my mother a much-deserved break. I didn't completely take over, but it was a huge relief to my family for me to be the interface with the hospice staff, plan my father's medication and when and how they should be given to him, answer the numerous phone calls that came in on an hourly basis, and to just be there with my father for those 2 months. I felt bad for my husband, Duane, as he was there with me the entire time. While there were some things he could do to help, there were many days when he felt helpless and frustrated and I hated that for him. On the other hand, there were many days that I never found time to brush my teeth, much less take a shower, but I didn't care. This was unchartered territory for me and what I thought was important was that my husband and I were there for my father, my mother, and the rest of my family.

So, to all of you who search the pages of this book, my hope is that you will find the answers that will assist you and the strength and encouragement to help you cope with the personal sadness or difficulties that you or a loved one may be experiencing. We have a common experience and perhaps I might be able to provide some additional insight into what you may be seeking.

This book is dedicated to the many people who have touched my heart in so many ways and provided encouragement and inspiration to live each day to the fullest and to never take life for granted. They have been there to cheer me on every step of the way—and there are still a lot of steps ahead of me.

Introduction

I owe a debt of gratitude and thanks to my husband, Duane, who has put up with the multitude of emotions from me over the last year. He has been my rock while I dealt with my father's death, left the safe environment of a successful career of almost 20 years, not to mention all of the experiences of starting my own business, all while trying to write (and finish) the second edition of *100 Questions & Answers About Brain Tumors*.

Dr. Stark-Vance, the second edition took a lot longer than we thought, but I have learned so much from you while writing this book. We spent many Sundays at your office writing, editing, and researching (while you were also taking calls from medical staff or making rounds). There were many times when I was ready to call it a day, but we kept going because you wanted to make sure that we provided the most updated medical information that brain cancer patients and caregivers were really looking for. It is no wonder why all of your patients and their families love you—it's because you care about them so much. You are much more than my neuro-oncologist; you are one of the most generous individuals I know. Over the past 9 years you have become a true friend and someone who has been there to provide medical (and personal) advice, support, and encouragement.

Authors always seem to acknowledge the support of family and now I know why. In the last year and a half, I have experienced many changes—some were painful, others were a leap of faith—but through it all, I still have my family and that means the world to me. My parents have always been my biggest fans and although my father passed away while I was writing this book, I am constantly reminded of his support and dedication to our family. My mother continues to be that voice I hear every day telling me, "you can do it" and "I'm so proud of you." I could never thank her enough for all the lessons, guidance, support, and encouragement that I can do anything.

My brothers, Dennis, Mark, and Steven, and my sister, Annemarie: it was growing up with you four that made me so competitive. You are the best.

I have tried to surround myself with great people—in life and in business. I have these people to thank: Jayne and Gil Romo, Kristy and Raymond Faus, Valerie Dillard, Tina and Don Fentem, Monsignor Henry Petter, Sue Davidson, and Karen and Bob Wucher. I thank each and every one of you for your inspiration, support, and encouragement over the past year and a half. You were there for me when I seemed to be at my wits' end and needed to vent, and you were there to celebrate my victories, too.

A big "thank you" goes to the editors and copywriters at Jones and Bartlett, who kept us on track for the last year and a half.

And to the many other people that I may have missed, please know how significant your comfort and inspiration has been to me.

Toffee Treats is ramping up for the 2009 holiday season and based on the feedback and progress so far, I believe we will have great success. I hope this piece of my story will inspire those of you who may fear that you will never be able to anything significant after surviving a brain tumor. Please don't be afraid to keep chasing your dreams.

While I still experience some fear and uncertainty, I know that God has a plan for me and I have been extremely blessed. So when I experience that fear and uncertainty, I try not to be afraid and realize that it is only change. My hope for you is that you will do the same. God bless you!

M.L. Dubay

PART ONE

The Basics

What is a brain tumor?

Why are there so many different types
of brain tumors?

Can any part of the brain have a tumor? Where in
the brain do most brain tumors occur? Are there
areas of the brain where it is more dangerous to
have a tumor?

More ...

1. What is a brain tumor?

The human brain is usually thought of as a single organ, a living computer that receives information from the senses and directs responses to our internal organs and muscles. Actually, the brain is only one part of the **central nervous system** (CNS), which also includes the spinal cord and the **meninges**, the three layers surrounding the brain and spinal cord. Like the other organs of the body, the CNS is composed of individual cells. These cells differ in their structure and function, but all have a normal function, directed by **deoxyribonucleic acid** (DNA), the internal genetic material of the cell nucleus. Occasionally, the genetic material develops a mutation or error that disrupts the function of the normal cell. If this abnormal cell continues to grow, divide, and produce more abnormal cells, the mass of abnormal cells may eventually become a visible tumor. In the brain, an enlarging mass of these abnormal cells that have "forgotten" their original function may disturb the surrounding normal cells in several ways (see **Figure 1**):

- The tumor may create pressure on a section of nearby normal brain, pushing the brain against the skull.
- The tumor may obstruct the flow of blood or spinal fluid circulating in the brain.
- The tumor may spread into the spinal fluid, creating more tumors in the brain and spinal cord.

The word "tumor" as used previously is not specified as **benign** or **malignant** (noncancerous and cancerous).

For some brain tumors, there is not a perfect distinction between these terms. Although benign tumors are often characterized as slow growing or unlikely to spread within the brain, some benign tumors cannot

---

Central nervous system (CNS)

Pertaining to the brain and spinal cord.

Meninges

Membranes covering the brain and spinal cord, consisting of the pia, arachnoid, and dura.

Deoxyribonucleic acid (DNA)

The genetic information in the cell nucleus, containing directions on cell growth, division, and function.

Benign

Not cancerous; not life threatening.

Malignant

Cancerous; cells that exhibit rapid, uncontrolled growth.

The Basics

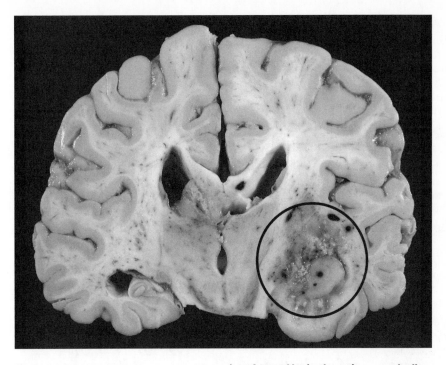

Figure 1   Tumors may create pressure on a section of normal brain, damaging normal cells in the surrounding area.

Source: Reproduced from Dr. K. Hatantaa, M.D., Neuropathologist, University of Texas Southwestern Medical School, Dallas, TX.

be removed surgically and therefore can cause severe disability and death. As a result, benign tumors can be dangerous because of their size and location, even though they may grow very slowly, displacing normal structures of the brain. Also, some types of benign tumors appear to develop further genetic damage over time and become even more rapidly growing masses, a process called **malignant transformation**. Malignant brain tumors tend to grow rapidly, damaging normal brain cells in the surrounding area. They may spread into other areas of the brain, spinal fluid, meninges, or spinal cord. Unlike malignant tumors of the breast, lung, colon, and other organs, malignant tumors of the brain rarely spread to other organs of the body.

Malignant transformation

The development of more destructive, invasive, or rapid growth in a previously benign or indolent tumor.

3

Despite their rapid growth and often destructive behavior, a few malignant tumors can also be cured because of their sensitivity to treatment. Over 100 different types of tumors originate in the brain, the spinal cord, or the meninges. Throughout this book, these tumors will be called **primary brain tumors**; however, many cancers originate in other organs of the body (e.g., the lung) and can spread through the bloodstream to the brain. When this occurs, the tumor formed is microscopically identical to the lung, even though it is now located in the brain. These tumors are called metastatic or **secondary brain tumors**. Some patients have brain metastases many years after the diagnosis of cancer. Some patients have brain metastases even before they know they have cancer.

2. Why are there so many different types of brain tumors?

To understand why there are so many types of brain tumors, it is necessary to learn some basic facts about normal brain cells. The **neurons** are cells that send electrical and chemical signals to other neurons. They perform the "work" of the nervous system. It is estimated that there are 1,000,000,000,000 (1 trillion) neurons, each with as many as 1,000 different connections to other neurons. The **glial cells**, which outnumber neurons nine to one, support the neurons. Some glial cells make **myelin**, an insulating sheath that allows neurons to conduct electrical signals at high speed. Some glial cells separate groups of neurons from each other, and some line the spinal fluid spaces of the brain. The major types of glial cells include **astrocytes**, **oligodendrocytes**, and **ependymal** cells.

How a normal cell becomes genetically damaged is not known, but the damage may cause the cell to divide repeatedly, producing a mass of cells. The most common brain tumor in adults is **astrocytoma**, which is not surprising, considering that the majority of glial cells in the brain are astrocytes. Similarly, abnormal oligodendrocytes that grow into a tumor become **oligodendrogliomas**, and abnormal ependymal cells become **ependymomas**. All of these tumors may be either benign (as the term is used previously here, slow growing) or malignant (fast growing, destructive). The names of many types of brain tumors are derived from their normal cell or tissue of origin, with the addition of the suffix "-oma." For example, tumors involving meninges are called **meningiomas**, tumors of the glial cells are called **gliomas**, and tumors involving Schwann cells are called Schwannomas.

3. Can any part of the brain have a tumor? Where in the brain do most brain tumors occur? Are there areas of the brain where it is more dangerous to have a tumor?

Both benign and malignant tumors can occur in all parts of the body, and the brain is no exception. The CNS includes the three major sections of the brain—the **cerebrum**, the **cerebellum**, the **brainstem**—and the spinal cord (**Figure 2**).

The cerebrum, the largest part of the brain, is divided into right and left **hemispheres**, which connect across the middle at the **corpus callosum**. The outer surface of the hemispheres, the **cortex**, is often called gray matter. It is slightly gray because of the dense population of cells packed into its convolutions (the ridges on the surface). At first glance, the cerebral hemispheres seem to have only a random collection of crevices and bulges, but there are deep folds or **fissures** that separate

Astrocytoma

A glioma that has developed from astrocytes.

Oligodendroglioma

Abnormal oligodendrocytes that grow into a tumor.

Ependymoma

Tumor that has developed from abnormal ependymal cells.

Meningiomas

A slow-growing tumor of the meninges.

Glioma

A tumor originating in the neuroglia of the brain or spinal cord.

Cerebrum

The largest area of the brain; divided into the right and left cerebral hemispheres.

The cerebrum, the largest part of the brain, is divided into right and left hemispheres, which connect across the middle at the corpus callosum.

The Basics

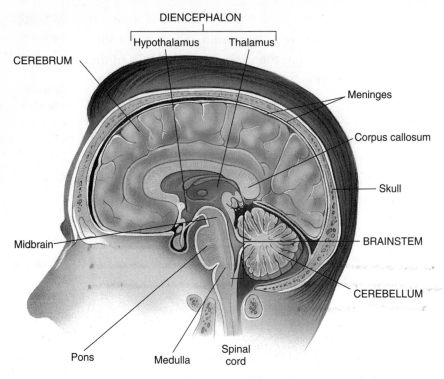

DIENCEPHALON

Hypothalamus   Thalamus

CEREBRUM

Meninges

Corpus callosum

Skull

Midbrain

BRAINSTEM

CEREBELLUM

Pons   Medulla   Spinal cord

Figure 2   The central nervous system, including the three major sections of the brain—the cerebrum, the cerebellum, the brainstem—and the spinal cord.

Cerebellum

Part of the brain located at the back of the head, under the cerebrum, and in back of the brainstem. Controls balance and coordination, affecting movements of the same side of the body.

Brainstem

That part of the central nervous system responsible for a number of "unconscious" activities, including breathing, heart rate, wakefulness, and sleep.

each hemisphere into lobes. Each cerebral hemisphere is subdivided into the **frontal lobe**, the **temporal lobe**, the **parietal lobe**, and the **occipital lobe**. Directly under the occipital lobe at the back of the head is the cerebellum, which is also divided into two hemispheres. The brainstem is a knob-like structure that is located in front of the cerebellum and under the cerebrum. The lower end of the brainstem is continuous with the spinal cord. Two elongated, curved openings in the center of each cerebral hemisphere, called the **lateral ventricles**, connect with two slit-like openings in the center of the brain, called the **third and fourth ventricles** (**Figure 3**). Spinal fluid is produced in the **choroid plexus**, sponge-like tissues in the lateral

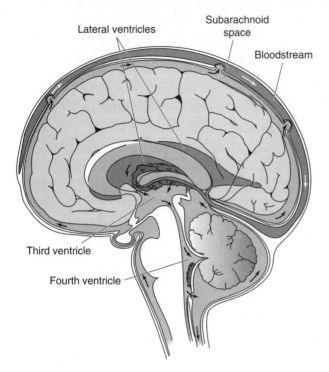

Figure 3   Two elongated, curved openings in each cerebral hemisphere, called the lateral ventricles, connect with two slit-like openings in the center of the brain, called the third and fourth ventricles.

Source: Illustration adapted from the American Brain Tumor Association.

ventricles. A tumor can occur in any of these parts of the brain, spinal cord, and meninges.

The symptoms of tumors vary with the location of the tumor. The **grade** influences how rapidly a tumor will cause symptoms. Grade refers to how much the tumor appears to resemble normal brain under the microscope. **Low-grade** tumors typically have few cells that are dividing at any one time. A **high-grade** tumor has a rapid growth rate, and the cells may appear disorganized and distorted. Tumors that are somewhere in between these two extremes are called **intermediate-grade** tumors.

Hemisphere

One of the two halves of the cerebrum or the cerebellum.

Corpus callosum

A prominent nerve fiber bundle in the center of the brain connecting the cerebral hemispheres.

Cortex

The outer surface of the cerebral hemispheres; often called the gray matter.

Fissures

The deep folds that separate each cerebral hemisphere into lobes.

Frontal lobe

The anterior (toward the face) area in the cerebral hemisphere involved in emotion, thought, reasoning, and behavior.

Temporal lobe

Area in the cerebral hemispheres that contain both the auditory and visual pathways and the interpretation of sounds and spoken language for long-term memory.

Parietal lobe

Area in the cerebral hemispheres that controls sensory and motor information.

The Basics

7

Occipital lobe

Area in the cerebral hemispheres that interpret visual images as well as the meaning of written words.

Lateral ventricles

The two elongated, curved openings in each cerebral hemisphere connecting with two slit-like openings in the center of the brain.

Third and fourth ventricles

Two spinal fluid-filled spaces in the center of the brain in communication with the lateral ventricles.

Choroid plexus

Two sponge-like tissues in the lateral ventricles that produce the spinal fluid.

Grade

The degree to which tumor tissue resembles normal tissue under the micro-scope. Tumors are classified as low grade if they are still very similar to nor-mal cells, high grade if they have a rapid growth rate with distorted or disor-ganized cells, or intermediate grade if they fall in between low and high grades.

The cerebral hemispheres direct motor function to the opposite site of the body, but the cerebellum, which coordinates movement, affects the same side of the body. For example, in most right-handed people, the left hemisphere controls speech as well as motor function to the right side of the body, and thus, the left hemisphere is considered the **dominant** hemisphere. Some left-handed people, however, are also considered left-hemisphere dominant because their speech center is located in the left hemisphere.

The frontal lobes of the cerebral hemispheres have four areas involved in personality, judgment, speech, and motor function. The prefrontal cortex, the portion of the brain behind the forehead, is involved in memory, planning, judgment, and personality. Below this area, near the temple, is the inferior frontal gyrus, which in the dominant hemisphere is called **Broca's area**. This area is involved in the production of spoken language. Another area, just behind the prefrontal cortex, is called the premotor area. This area controls the initiation and sequencing of voluntary motor movements. Finally, at an area that marks the border of the frontal and parietal lobes, the **precentral gyrus**, is a large area, the primary motor cortex, which gives rise to voluntary movements to the opposite side of the body. Interestingly, this area has been mapped to reveal specific areas corresponding to the foot and lower extremity near the top of the brain, and the face, lips, and tongue near the bottom.

The parietal lobes control the localization and discrimi-nation of sensory information. In the dominant hemi-sphere, the parietal lobe also discriminates between right and left and is involved in mental calculation and written language. The nondominant hemisphere of the parietal lobe processes awareness of the spatial orientation of the body.

The temporal lobes contain both auditory and visual pathways and interpret sounds and spoken language for long-term memory. The temporal lobes also contain the **limbic system**, which is involved in learning and the emotional content of memories.

The occipital lobes interpret and process visual information.

The cerebellum controls balance and coordination, affecting movements of the same side of the body.

The brainstem is responsible for a number of "unconscious" activities, including breathing, heart rate, swallowing, wakefulness, and sleep. Many of the **cranial nerves**, the nerves that provide motor and sensory function to the eyes, mouth, tongue, neck, and shoulders arise from the brainstem. The brainstem is continuous with the spinal cord, separated by the **foramen magnum**, the large hole at the base of the skull.

The cerebral hemispheres make up the largest mass of the CNS, and most of the primary brain tumors affecting adults occur in this area. In children, primary brain tumors more often affect the cerebellum and brain-. stem. Spinal cord tumors are relatively uncommon in both age groups.

The brainstem and cranial nerves are surrounded by the base of the skull, which has numerous small openings for the blood vessels and nerves that travel to and from the brain; however, the space within the skull is limited. An expanding tumor that exerts pressure on

The Basics

Low grade
Tumors that have few cells dividing at any one time, often resembling normal tissue.

High grade
Tumor that has a rapid growth rate; the cells may appear disorganized and distorted.

Intermediate grade
Tumors that have features of aggressiveness and growth characteristics between low- and high-grade tumors.

Dominant
Ruling or controlling. The cerebral hemisphere that controls speech formation is referred to as the dominant hemisphere.

Broca's area
An area in the frontal lobe of the brain that is associated with speech.

Precentral gyrus
An area of the brain that contains the primary motor cortext, which controls voluntary muscle movement.

Limbic system

A group of deep brain structures that are associated with emotions, behavior, learning, and memory.

Cranial nerves

Nerves that arise from the base of the brain or the brainstem that provide sensory and motor function to the eyes, nose, ears, tongue, and face.

Foramen magnum

A large hole at the base of the skull; it serves as the boundary between the brainstem and the spinal cord.

Computed tomography (CT)

Computerized series of X-rays that create a detailed cross-sectional image of the body.

Magnetic resonance imaging (MRI)

A radiographic study based on the acquisition of anatomical information using resonance from atoms in a strong magnetic field.

the brainstem may affect consciousness, heart rate, and breathing. Tumors in this area are also more difficult to remove without injuring the normal brain structures and blood vessels. Although all tumors can cause symptoms, tumors that directly or indirectly affect the brainstem are some of the most difficult and dangerous to treat.

4. How common are brain tumors? Is it true that brain tumors are more common in children than in adults?

About 1.2 million adults in the United States are diagnosed with cancer every year, and of those, 52,200 will have a primary brain tumor. Almost half of primary brain tumors are malignant. Primary brain tumors account for only about 2.3% of all cancer deaths in adults, compared with about 28.6% caused by lung cancer and 7.2% caused by breast cancer. The incidences of breast cancer and lung cancer are very high, but similar to lung cancer, many brain tumors are found only after they have become symptomatic, when the opportunity for successful treatment and cure may be lower. Although the 5-year survival for brain tumors patients has increased since 1975, it is still only 34%, and for some of the most common primary brain tumors, the 5-year survival is much less.

The incidence of brain tumors was noted to increase after both **computed tomography** (CT) and **magnetic resonance imaging** (MRI) scans became widely available in the 1980s. Before the availability of neuroimaging, many patients were assumed to have other neurological disorders such as stroke or dementia. Even today, however, it is likely that thousands of people have small, benign tumors such as meningiomas that are not discovered because they are not symptomatic.

Such tumors are frequently discovered when the patient undergoes an MRI for another reason. These "incidental" findings are not reported in national databases; therefore, even though meningiomas are the most common primary brain tumors in adults, their true incidence may never be known.

The incidence of both primary and metastatic brain tumors increases in patients with age. Many people are unaware that brain tumors are the second leading cause of cancer death in men up to age 39 years and the fifth leading cause of cancer death in women ages 20 to 39 years. The median age of diagnosis of all primary brain tumors is 57 years. Survival in the over-75 age group is poor, with only 5% of patients achieving 5-year survival.

The incidence of both primary and metastatic brain tumors increases in patients with age.

The most common cancers that metastasize to the brain, spinal cord, and spinal fluid are lung cancer (particularly small cell lung cancer), breast cancer, melanoma, and kidney cancer. Interestingly, although prostate cancer is the most common cancer in men, brain metastases from prostate cancer are rare. Because of the combined number of cancer patients with metastatic disease to the CNS, metastatic brain tumors outnumber primary brain tumors by at least four to one. Although survival data in **metastatic tumors** are more difficult to obtain, the development of metastatic disease to the brain or spinal cord clearly results in a shortened survival for most patients. Obviously, the disability and death that result from primary and metastatic tumors exceed that of *all* other cancers.

Metastatic tumors
Cancer that has spread outside of the organ or structure in which it arose to another area of the body.

In the United States, brain tumors account for about 23% of all cancers in children (about 3,750 cases). Only leukemia is a more common cause of cancer-related

The Basics

death in children less than 20 years old. Although meningiomas are more common in adults, gliomas are the most common type of tumor in children. Gliomas may be either benign or malignant, but the benign, slow-growing variety is more common in the pediatric age group; therefore, the 5-year survival in the under-20 group is almost twice that of adults, 66%.

Further information on the incidence and survival related to brain tumors is available from the Central Brain Tumor Registry of the United States at www.cbtrus.org.

5. What causes a brain tumor?

Because there are so many different types of brain tumors, each originating from the different types of cells within the brain, spinal cord, or meninges, it is impossible to determine a cause for most brain tumors. There are, however, known risk factors for the development of some types of tumors.

Cigarette smoking has not been clearly associated with an increased risk for the development of primary brain tumors, but smoking is an important cause of metastatic brain tumors, particularly those that originate from lung cancer. Of the 213,000 lung cancer patients diagnosed each year in the United States, about one-third—more than 70,000 people!—will develop one or more tumors in the brain.

Some primary brain tumors affect men more commonly than women and vice versa, but the reasons for these differences are not known. Some studies suggest that workers in certain occupations have a higher incidence of brain tumors. It has been known for several years that workers in the petrochemical industry have a higher incidence of brain tumors, and exposure to vinyl chloride has been recognized as a CNS carcinogen; however, for many of the occupations reported to have an increased risk of CNS tumors, such as business managers and messengers, no known environmental exposure has been identified.

Table 1 lists occupations that have been associated with an increased risk of brain tumors. The increased risk is expressed as an odds ratio. The odds ratio is found by dividing the odds of being in a specific occupation and having a brain tumor by the odds of being in the occupation but not having a brain tumor. For many occupations studied, there was no known exposure to a potential cancer-causing chemical. Some researchers have suggested that patients with professional or highly paid jobs have better access to medical

Table 1   Occupations Associated with Increased Risk of Brain Tumors

Occupation	Odds Ratio	Comments
Statisticians	3.72	Study from New Zealand, 1989
Livestock farmers	2.59	Exposure to animal disease
Truck drivers	6.65	Specifically glioma
Utility workers	13.1	
Printers, publishers	2.8	
Brick masons	2.5	
French farmers	1.25	Possibly related to pesticide use in vineyards
Petroleum workers	2.9	Not all studies show increased risk
Electrical workers	2.8	Risk increased with exposure to electromagnetic fields
Clergymen	3.8	

care, which may result in a greater number of brain tumors diagnosed; however, interestingly, in Sweden, where there is universal access to free medical care, some occupations are still observed to have a higher risk of brain tumors. These include medical professionals, biologists, agricultural research scientists, and dentists.

Patients who have previously had radiation therapy to the brain, skull, or scalp are at risk for developing brain tumors many years later.

Patients who have previously had **radiation therapy** to the brain, skull, or scalp are at risk for developing brain tumors many years later. This is particularly important because of the risk of developing a second tumor after successful treatment for a brain tumor in childhood. There is no known intervention that can reduce the risk of developing a radiation-related tumor. Several studies have investigated other sources of radiation, such as electromagnetic fields, power lines, and cell phones; however, studies have not yet proven that these sources cause brain tumors.

Radiation therapy

Treatment that uses high-dose X-rays or other high-energy rays to kill cancer cells and shrink tumors.

Head injury, hair dye, and drug use have also been studied, but it has not been shown conclusively that these factors cause primary brain tumors. Food additives and preservatives and chemicals in drinking water have been studied in a number of countries. For example, eating preserved, smoked, or pickled meat and fish appears to correlate with an increased risk of brain tumors. In addition, two studies have shown that the risk of brain tumor decreases when individuals eat more fruits and vegetables; however, other studies of dietary influence on the development of brain tumors have been inconclusive.

In summary, although many factors have been studied for a possible link to the development of primary brain tumors, few are considered definite risk factors.

6. Are brain tumors inherited?

Some genetic diseases are clearly associated with the development of specific brain tumors. Fortunately, most of these are rare. Whereas only about 5% of brain tumor patients have a family member with the same or a very similar brain tumor, about 19% of all brain tumor patients have a close family member with another type of cancer. This suggests that the tendency to develop genetic damage that causes abnormal cell growth may be inherited, but the tendency to develop a specific type of tumor may not be inherited.

Table 2 lists genetic syndromes that have been associated with brain tumors. A brain tumor may contain one or multiple mutations, but that does not mean that the abnormal gene containing the mutation will be inherited by the patient's children. Only those abnormal genes that are present in the reproductive cells (eggs and sperm) are inherited. In many of the syndromes listed, more than one type of cancer has been described. In **Turcot's syndrome**, for example, all patients who inherit the gene will develop colon cancer if untreated. Because of more widespread genetic testing, many families who are affected by one of the genetic syndromes shown in Table 2 are aware of their increased cancer risk.

Sporadic mutations (those that develop spontaneously and are not present in the reproductive cells) account for more than 95% of all brain tumors; however, some of the same mutations described in inherited brain tumors also occur in tumors arising spontaneously. The *p53* mutation, for example, is found in over 50% of all human cancers. For reasons that are unclear, younger patients with glioblastoma are more likely to have a *p53* mutation than older patients.

Whereas only about 5% of brain tumor patients have a family member with the same or a very similar brain tumor, about 19% of all brain tumor patients have a close family member with another type of cancer.

Turcot's syndrome

An inherited condition associated with colon polyps and brain tumors.

The Basics

Table 2   Genetic Syndromes Associated with Brain Tumors

Syndrome	Chromosomal Abnormality	Gene	CNS Tumors Associated with Abnormality
Multiple Endocrine Neoplasia Type 1	11	*MEN-1*	Pituitary adenoma
Neurofibromatosis 1	17	*NF1*	Neurofibromas, optic nerve glioma, meningioma, nerve sheath tumors
Tuberous Sclerosis	9, 16	*TSC1/TSC2*	Subependymal giant cell astrocytoma
Von Hippel-Lindau	3	*VHL*	Hemangioblastoma
Li-Fraumeni	17	*p53*	Glioma
Gorlin's Syndrome	9	*Ptc*	Medulloblastoma
Turcot's Syndrome	5	*APC*	Astrocytoma, glioblastoma, medulloblastoma
Cowden's Disease	10	*PTEN*	Dysplastic gangliocytoma of cerebellum
Pallister-Hall Syndrome	7	*Gli3*	Hypothalamic hamartoma
Rubinstein-Taybi Syndrome	16	*CBP*	Medulloblastoma, oligodendroglioma, neuroblastoma, meningioma
Familial Retinoblastoma Syndrome	13	*Rb*	Retinoblastoma, glioma, meningioma, pineoblastoma

M.L.'s comment:

It was June 28, 2000, when I found out that I had a brain tumor. That day was supposed to be just like any other day, but when my alarm went off I woke up feeling like I had the flu, and I just wanted to go back to sleep. I remember that I didn't sleep well the night before. I just kept tossing and turning. I felt like I never really went to sleep all night. I hadn't ever had a migraine, much less a headache, but when I finally did get up I knew something wasn't right.

It was 6 a.m., and I was in the shower getting ready to go to work. I remember feeling just awful, as if I were going to faint. My husband, Duane, was out of town, so I couldn't ask him for help, and he wasn't there to see if I was acting strangely. When I got out of the shower all I could think about was how tired I was and that I wanted to go back to bed. I just thought that I needed more sleep because I had worked late at the office the night before.

A close friend of mine took me to the emergency room that was just a few blocks away. Once I was in the emergency room, everything became a blur! Later, I was told that I underwent a series of tests, including a CT scan and an MRI. After many tests and lots of questions, the doctors determined that I had an abnormality on the left side of my brain. I was admitted to the hospital and was started on antiseizure medication. The doctors were concerned that I may have had a mild seizure the night before, and they wanted to prevent a possible recurrence.

My husband arrived at the hospital later that day, and that is when the doctors told us that the tests had revealed a mass in the left frontal lobe. It appeared to be a "glial-type" brain tumor; however, they indicated that the tumor was located in an area of my brain where it could be surgically removed.

At this point, it was time to let my family know what had happened to me over the last several hours. My husband immediately called my parents in Knoxville, Tennessee. Although this was extremely shocking news, my father, a retired orthopedic surgeon, and my mother, a former Navy nurse, understood exactly what they had been told. My parents then informed the rest of my family (three older brothers and one older sister), all of whom live in Knoxville. I'm the youngest of five children, and I live 1,000 miles away from the rest of the family. I can imagine how difficult it must have been for them.

I was kept in the hospital for a few days. Then I was allowed to go home to "enjoy" the 4th of July weekend. I returned to the hospital the morning of July 6th so that my neurosurgeon could remove the mass in my brain. For the week or so between diagnosis and surgery, I really don't remember too many details. I was probably in some state of shock; however, when my neurosurgeon told me that I had a brain tumor, the reality set in. That was when it became very clear to me that the world as I had known it had changed forever, and my journey of living with a brain tumor began.

Update as of July 2008:

When Dr. Virginia Stark-Vance and I started working on the second edition of this book in early 2008, I didn't think I'd have much to add in terms of an update on my condition. After all, I had been cancer-free for 7 years and was looking forward to celebrating my 8-year anniversary over the 4th of July weekend of 2008.

My husband, Duane, and I had planned an extended vacation and decided to spend the week of the 4th of July holiday in Hilton Head Island, South Carolina with my family. From there, we were going to spend a few days in Charleston, South Carolina, just the two of us before heading back to Dallas. We had celebrated our 15th wedding anniversary in June and wanted to have a few days by ourselves, so we made plans to stay at this beautiful bed and breakfast and see the sites of this historical city.

*We were excited about our trip to Charleston because nei-
ther of us had ever been there. The first night we arrived
in Charleston, which is only a couple of hours drive from
Hilton Head, we decided to go on one of the highly
acclaimed "Ghosts and Graveyards" tour. It didn't start
until 10:00 p.m., but we didn't care. . . . We were on vacation!!! I think we thought we really were going to see some
ghosts, but unfortunately, we did not.*

*Nevertheless, the next day we spent most of the day taking
in the history of how the Civil War began at Fort Sumter.
I remember it being especially hot and humid that day, but
what else would you expect for July in South Carolina? We
had a great day and even more fun that evening as we
experienced the sites and sounds of this beautiful city.*

*The next day, Duane wanted to explore some more Civil
War history, and I decided to do some shopping on my own
in the famous upper King Street section of Charleston since
we were leaving the next day. We decided to meet back at
our bed and breakfast later that afternoon so that we
would have plenty of time to enjoy our last evening in
Charleston.*

*Unfortunately, that was the last time I saw Duane for a
few days. . . .*

*Duane dropped me off in the heart of the city so that I
could get in a few hours of "power shopping," and he headed
off to Patriots Point to check out some of the aircraft and
ships used during the Civil War.*

*The first shop that I went into was a neat little boutique. I
was walking around with several pieces of clothing in my
hand, and I remember hearing this faint little voice in the
back of my mind saying, "I'm not sure I know how to buy*

these clothes," and put them back on the rack. A minute or so later, I thought, "Wait a second, I do know how to buy these clothes." So I went back over and picked them back up off the rack. This is the point where it all went fuzzy and the following is what my husband told me.

Evidently, a store sales associate came up to me and asked if she could start a dressing room for me. She told Duane that I made some weird noise and just fell to the floor and immediately started seizing. That was the first of three grand mal seizures that I would experience that afternoon! I feel so fortunate that the sales associates were trained in first aid and knew to clear people and items away from the immediate area around me. They called 911.

Once Duane arrived at the hospital, they told him that I had been placed in the intensive care unit because I was having trouble breathing on my own. They had me on a respirator (or breathing machine) with a tube down my throat with lots of other needles and tubes sticking out of both of my arms. I was completely out of it, as they had given me significant amounts of Dilantin to stop the seizures.

The medical staff informed Duane of what had happened, and he provided all of the details of my medical history over the last 8 years. To say that he was pretty shaken up when he saw me is an understatement, but he managed to keep it together—at least for a while.

My mother and sister-in-law arrived the next day from Knoxville, Tennessee. Unsure of my condition, my mother was prepared to come back to Dallas just in case she needed to help Duane take care of me. Fortunately, that wasn't necessary.

I spent 3 days in the ICU, but I don't remember any of them—in hindsight, that's probably a good thing. I do remember that after an MRI and CT scan, the doctors did not find any sign of recurring tumor.

We returned to Dallas, and I took the next few weeks off, as I was very tired and need to rest and regain my strength. Because I had been on a respirator for 3 days, it was difficult for me to talk for a few days. The tubes had irritated my throat, so my breathing and talking was more labored than normal.

Within the next couple of weeks, I made sure to do all of the proper follow-up with my local doctors. I had an EEG, and thankfully, the results came back normal. One change I did make was to get back on my antiseizure medication.

To this day, the only explanation that I've been given is that a seizure can occur under three main conditions: lack of food, lack of sleep, and/or lack of medication. Well, I would have to say that all three of those conditions were present when I had my seizures. Per my doctor's approval, I had been able to discontinue my antiseizure medication 4 years prior. I would also imagine that the extreme heat and humidity in Charleston coupled with inconsistent eating and sleeping habits over the previous 10-day period may have also contributed to the situation.

Interestingly, my neurosurgeon had told me that the likelihood of my having a seizure was 2% to 3%. With those odds, I probably shouldn't consider playing the lottery.

After I went back to work I was committed to taking things a little slower for a few more weeks, per my doctor's advice. Everyone was so shocked to hear what had happened to me. Many didn't even know that I was a brain cancer survivor, so to hear about this situation literally left some of them speechless.

It is easy to get complacent when a certain period of time passes with no symptoms. I have to admit that I was feeling that I had beaten brain cancer 8 years before, and then "POW!" something happened to remind me that I still need to be careful. In a situation like this, we are reminded of what is really important in life. We have to listen to our bodies and remember that while our work and activities are important, our health is even more important.

PART TWO

Diagnosis and Pathology

What are the symptoms of brain tumors? Do all brain tumors cause headaches?

Why does every doctor I see ask me so many questions about my symptoms, my previous illnesses, and my family history?

What is a neurological examination?

More . . .

Although more than 99% of adults who suffer from headaches do not have a brain tumor, about half of all brain tumor patients complain of a headache at the time of diagnosis.

7. What are the symptoms of brain tumors? Do all brain tumors cause headaches?

Brain tumors may be discovered even when they do not cause any symptoms because brain scans are commonly performed in emergency rooms after head trauma; however, the nature and duration of symptoms are important clues to the location of the tumor and sometimes may even suggest the type of tumor present (**Figure 4**).

It is estimated that every day 10 million people in the United States suffer from headaches. Although more than 99% of adults who suffer from headaches do not

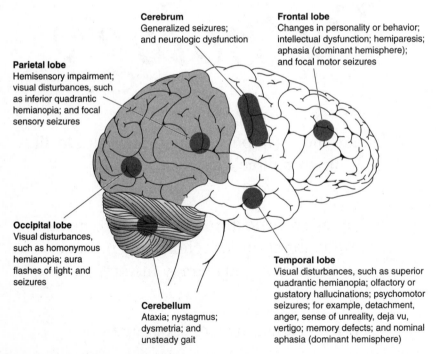

Parietal lobe
Hemisensory impairment; visual disturbances, such as inferior quadrantic hemianopia; and focal sensory seizures

Cerebrum
Generalized seizures; and neurologic dysfunction

Frontal lobe
Changes in personality or behavior; intellectual dysfunction; hemiparesis; aphasia (dominant hemisphere); and focal motor seizures

Occipital lobe
Visual disturbances, such as homonymous hemianopia; aura flashes of light; and seizures

Cerebellum
Ataxia; nystagmus; dysmetria; and unsteady gait

Temporal lobe
Visual disturbances, such as superior quadrantic hemianopia; olfactory or gustatory hallucinations; psychomotor seizures; for example, detachment, anger, sense of unreality, deja vu, vertigo; memory defects; and nominal aphasia (dominant hemisphere)

Figure 4   Signs and symptoms of intracranial tumors.

Source: Adapted from *Coping with Neurologic Disorders,* c. 1982, Intermed Communications, Inc.

have a brain tumor, about half of all brain tumor patients complain of a headache at the time of diagnosis. Because children seem to suffer headaches less frequently than adults, a child under 10 who complains of headache should always raise the suspicion of a brain tumor.

The incidence of headache in brain tumor patients is related to both the growth rate and location of the tumor. Slow-growing tumors are more likely to cause seizures than headaches, whereas faster growing tumors may cause headaches as an initial symptom. Tumors that obstruct the flow of spinal fluid are more commonly associated with a headache and nausea.

Headaches associated with brain tumors do not always follow a clear, progressive pattern of increasing severity. The headache may be worse in the morning or interfere with sleep, or it may occur with bending, lifting, or exercise. Headaches caused by brain tumors may be relieved with medications used to treat migraine or tension headaches, or even over-the-counter drugs such as acetaminophen (Tylenol) or aspirin.

Other frequent symptoms noted by brain tumor patients include nausea and vomiting, visual problems, seizures, weakness, confusion, imbalance, depression, and fatigue. It is not unusual for family members to note subtle changes in an individual's personality. These changes may be difficult for a doctor to detect unless she is very familiar with the patient. **Neurological deficit** refers to partial or complete loss of muscle strength, sensation, or other brain functions that may become more pronounced with fatigue. Almost all patients with brain tumors exhibit at least

Neurological deficit

Partial or complete loss of muscle strength, sensation, or other brain functions; may be temporary or permanent.

some neurological deficit at the time of diagnosis, although it may be very subtle.

8. Why does every doctor I see ask me so many questions about my symptoms, my previous illnesses, and my family history?

Medical history

A detailed accounting by the patient that helps a physician to determine the length and severity of an illness as well as previous personal and family health history.

Nonlocalizing

Symptoms not confined, limited, or contained to a specific area; may be attributed to other illnesses, depression, or stress. Examples include fatigue, lack of concentration, or nausea.

Localizing

Symptoms suggesting that a specific area of the nervous system is involved, for example, speech disturbance, weakness of one side of the body, or loss of vision.

Edema

Swelling or fluid build-up.

A detailed **medical history** is extremely important to a doctor. It helps to determine the length and severity of an illness. Most brain tumor patients have symptoms that may have initially been attributed to other illnesses, depression, or stress. For example, it is common for patients to complain of fatigue, a lack of concentration, or nausea. These **nonlocalizing** symptoms may be easily dismissed by patients and their doctors. **Localizing** symptoms, such as speech disturbance, weakness of one side of the body, or seizures, are more likely to raise the suspicion of a neurological problem. In addition, the history may guide the physician to the type of tests ordered.

A patient who complains of a severe headache, for example, may or may not need an emergency computed tomography (CT) scan of the brain. Perhaps the patient has a history of migraine headaches for years and has had a normal CT scan in the past. Perhaps the patient fell from a ladder and briefly lost consciousness. Perhaps the patient has had escalating headaches for several weeks that are now unbearable. The doctor must decide, based on the history and physical examination, whether other tests are in order. Most commonly, a CT scan of the brain will be obtained for these patients to evaluate for the presence of blood within the brain, any distortion of the normal shape and size of the brain structures, and any **edema** (swelling) of the brain. Occasionally, however, a very small tumor or subtle abnormality will not be seen on CT, and other tests such as magnetic resonance imaging (MRI) (see Part Three) will be required.

If a tumor is revealed on the scan, the doctor can sometimes estimate the type of tumor and its growth rate from details in the patient's history. The doctor will also determine whether the patient has a previous history of cancer because of the possibility of a metastatic, rather than a primary, brain tumor. The doctor may also note whether there is a family history of cancer or brain tumor and whether the patient has other inherited conditions that may impact on the patient's care, such as bleeding disorders, diabetes, and heart disease. All of these factors will be noted before referral to a specialist, and then the specialist will ask the same questions all over again! Not surprisingly, every physician will want to make sure to be familiar with all of the details of the patient's case and will want to verify any previous records that the patient has submitted.

9. What is a neurological examination?

The part of the physical examination called the **neurological examination** actually begins before the patient is aware of it. From the time the patient walks into the examination room, the doctor observes the patient's balance, rhythm, and coordination. During the history, the doctor will observe the patient's speech patterns—whether there is hesitation, difficulty finding words, misuse of words, or slurring of words. Even the patient's eye movements can suggest whether there is a neurological problem.

A neurological examination may be as simple as testing strength, sensation, and coordination in the emergency

Neurological examination

Part of the physical examination testing general intellectual function, speech, motor function, memory, sensation, reflexes, and cranial nerve functions.

A neurological examination may be as simple as testing strength, sensation, and coordination in the emergency room setting or testing a series of more complex physical and memory tasks in the neurologist's office.

room setting or testing a series of more complex physical and memory tasks in the neurologist's office. A complete neurological examination evaluates the following:

1. Appearance and behavior: Is the patient behaving appropriately for the situation?
2. Standing and walking: Is there imbalance or jerking of movement?
3. Level of consciousness: Is the patient fully alert?
4. Orientation to time and place: Does the patient know the year, month, day, and where he is at that moment?
5. General intellectual function: Does the patient misinterpret clues from the environment or seem confused?
6. Memory: Can the patient remember three unrelated words for 5 minutes?
7. Speech: Can the patient understand and respond to spoken language?
8. Cranial nerve functions:
   a. Can the patient smell?
   b. Can the patient see clearly with each eye separately?
   c. Can the patient look up and down and raise the eyelids?
   d. Can the patient look down and toward the nose?
   e. Can the patient open the jaw? Does the patient have sensation on both sides of the face?
   f. Can the patient move the eyes to the right and left?
   g. Can the patient close the eyes tightly and smile symmetrically?
   h. Can the patient hear with each ear?

   i. Can the patient swallow?

   j. Can the patient shrug his shoulders?

   k. Can the patient stick out his tongue?

9. Motor function: Does the patient have normal muscle power in all extremities?

10. Reflexes: Are the patient's reflexes symmetrical?

11. Coordination: Can the patient touch his finger to his nose rapidly and accurately?

12. Sensation: Can the patient perceive light touch, temperature, position, vibration, and pain?

Some doctors use the **Mini-Mental Status Examination**, which is a set of questions and tasks that can be easily administered in the office or hospital setting. The Mini-Mental Status Examination tests orientation, memory, calculation, language, and figure drawing on a 30-point scale. The test results are kept with the patient's chart to determine whether a change has occurred in the patient's status over time.

Mini-Mental Status Examination

A brief verbal and written examination that tests orientation, memory, calculation, language, and figure drawing on a 30-point scale.

Patients sometimes object that the neurological examination is "stupid," "a waste of time," or "insulting." Nothing could be further from the truth! What could possibly be more important than verifying that the most important organ that we possess is functioning correctly? Clearly, you would not buy a car without taking it for a test drive and checking the performance of its engine. Similarly, your doctor should not be expected to merely look at you and know that you can tell time, count backward from 100, or remember three objects for 5 minutes. It is important to remember that severely demented patients may look and speak perfectly normally— until someone asks them what year it is. It should be clear that you want your physician, each and every time that you are asked, to have a very complete record that your brain is functioning normally.

10. After my surgery, my surgeon told me that I have a brain tumor but says that he cannot tell me more about it until the pathology report is completed. What is a pathology report, and why is it so important?

Because there are many different types of brain tumors, your surgeon wants to give you as much detailed information as possible about the kind of tumor you have and the treatment you may need. The doctor cannot do that until a **pathologist** examines the **biopsy** taken at surgery. Some tumors can be evaluated within a few minutes using thin slices of frozen tumor; however, most tumors require processing over a period of several hours. During processing, the water is removed from the specimen. Eventually, tiny pieces of the tumor are embedded in paraffin wax. These small slabs of paraffin-embedded tissue are thinly sliced, placed on microscope slides, and stained with special chemicals that color the cell proteins and deoxyribonucleic acid (DNA). These are called permanent sections, and their detail provides the pathologist with the most complete information about the tumor.

The pathologist provides information about the cells that make up the tumor and identifies whether the cells are native to the brain (a primary tumor) or if they have spread to the brain from another location in the body (a metastatic tumor). The pathologist determines whether the tumor is benign or malignant. The growth rate, or **proliferation index**, can

Pathologist

A physician trained to examine and evaluate cells, tissue, and organs for the presence of disease.

Biopsy

Surgical removal of a small piece of tissue or a tumor for microscopic examination.

Proliferation index

A measurement of the growth and division rate of cells obtained from a biopsy specimen, using special stains.

also be obtained from the biopsy specimen using special stains.

In some cases, the pathologist may confer with other colleagues or send the slides to a **neuropathologist**, a pathologist who specializes in the diseases of the nervous system. Difficult cases may take several days of study to determine the exact nature of the tumor. The final diagnosis is written in the pathology report (see the section "How to Read Your Pathology Report" on pages 38–39). The importance of this document cannot be overstated. Determining eligibility for clinical trials, the need for further treatment such as radiation therapy or chemotherapy, and the eligibility for insurance or disability benefits are a few of the reasons that the pathology report is the single most important document to the brain tumor patient. Also, you will want to know the correct name of your tumor if you decide to research your treatment options. Because the *exact* name of the tumor is so important (a glioma is not the same as a glioblastoma, and a pituitary adenoma is not the same as a pituitary carcinoma), ask your doctor for a copy of the pathology report. If you have trouble understanding the terminology, do not hesitate to ask your physician to underline the name of the tumor and explain any specific terms used to describe your tumor. You must also understand whether it is a primary or metastatic tumor, whether it is benign or malignant, and whether any other studies have been completed or are pending. For example, it is not unusual to have further testing for genetic mutations, specific growth factor receptors, and drug resistance on brain tumor specimens. As you learn more about your specific tumor and your treatment options, you will understand how your physician uses these results to guide your therapy (**Table 3**).

Diagnosis and Pathology

Neuropathologist
Pathologist specializing in the diagnosis of diseases of the peripheral and central nervous systems.

If you have trouble understanding the terminology, do not hesitate to ask your physician to underline the name of the tumor and explain any specific terms used to describe your tumor.

Table 3   Common Types of Primary Brain Tumors in Adults and Children

CNS Tumors in Adults		CNS Tumors in Children	
Glioblastoma multiforme and anaplastic astrocytoma	35%	Low-grade gliomas and brain-stem glioma	44%
Meningiomas	25%	Primitive neuroectodermal tumors (PNET) and medulloblastoma	24%
Low grade gliomas and brainstem gliomas	12%	Ependymoma	10%
Pituitary adenoma	10%	Pineal region tumors, including germinoma	6%
Acoustic neuroma	7%	Glioblastoma and anaplastic astrocytoma	4%
Other	11%	Other	12%

M.L.'s comment:

I had no idea how important the pathology report was. Although the actual report wasn't reviewed with me, my neurosurgeon did discuss the specifics of it. He indicated that the pathology report revealed that I had an anaplastic oligo-dendroglioma. However, after my neurosurgeon received the analysis, he sent it back to be retested because he thought that what he removed looked like something other than an oligo. Nevertheless, the test came back again with the same result.

Clearly, an accurate diagnosis is extremely important to your medical team because the recommended treatment hinges on the interpretation of the pathology report. A copy of the pathology report was one of the first documents that I had to send to my disability advisor after my surgery so that I could apply for temporary disability.

Since my diagnosis, I have been surprised to talk with other brain tumor patients who do not know the type of tumor they have. I have learned that in some countries it is unusual for patients to receive a copy of their pathology report (or any other reports) from their physicians. I'm glad I had a copy of

*my report when my husband and I began researching infor-
mation about my tumor because I knew treatment would
hinge on the pathologist's final diagnosis.*

11. What are the most common types of primary brain tumors?

Table 3 lists the most common types of primary brain
tumors in children and adults. In both children and
adults, gliomas are the most common type of tumor
(see Color Plates 1 and 2); however, adults have a
higher proportion of malignant, or high-grade, glioma,
and children have a higher proportion of slower growing, low-grade, glioma. In addition, adults tend to have
tumors of the cerebral hemispheres, and children more
commonly have tumors of the cerebellum and brainstem. Some tumor types, such as primitive neuroectodermal tumor, medulloblastoma, and ependymoma,
are much more common in children; meningiomas are
much more common in adults. In fact, it is not unusual
to find a small, benign meningioma in a patient who is
symptomatic from a more aggressively growing glioma
or metastatic tumor. Of the metastatic brain tumors,
lung cancer is the most frequent primary source, but
breast cancer, kidney cancer, and melanoma are also
common primaries.

12. The surgeon explained to me that I have a fast-growing type of tumor, but I think my symptoms have been present for a long time. Is this possible? Should I get a second opinion from another pathologist to make sure that the diagnosis is correct? How do I do this?

You may have a slow-growing tumor that evolved into
a faster-growing type. The pathologist may have only
seen the faster growing component in the tumor specimen

studied. Not surprisingly, the treatment recommended for patients with such mixed tumors depends on the more aggressive component.

A second review of your pathology slides can be helpful, but pathologists often confer with others in the same hospital or send the slides to a colleague for further review. It is possible that your slides were reviewed by a handful of pathologists before the final report was issued. Nevertheless, an additional review—even if the same pathologist does it—may be helpful if you provide clinical information, such as what type of symptoms you have and how long your symptoms have persisted. It is also beneficial if you forward a copy of your MRI to the pathologist.

Getting a second opinion about your pathology slides is particularly important if a different diagnosis will have an impact on your treatment and prognosis.

Getting a second opinion about your pathology slides is particularly important if a different diagnosis will have an impact on your treatment and prognosis. You may ask your surgeon whether he recommends sending the slides to another laboratory or research center that specializes in brain tumors. If you plan to participate in a clinical trial, another review of your pathology slides by a neuropathologist associated with the trial is often required and will be arranged by the investigator directing the trial.

13. My doctor says that my tumor has a low proliferation index and that I may not need treatment right away. What is the proliferation index, and how does it determine my treatment?

The proliferation index is determined by testing some of the brain tumor sample using a special stain for MIB-1 or Ki-67. The proliferation index is the number of cells involved in the process of cell division (the process that produces new tumor cells) in relationship to the total number of cells. Slow-growing tumors have few dividing cells, meaning that they have a low proliferation index (sometimes less than 1%). Tumors that grow more rapidly may have proliferation indices exceeding 20%. Tumors with a low proliferation index grow relatively slowly, and even without treatment, they may not appear to have observable growth on an MRI over many months. Tumors with a high proliferation index may double in size within days or weeks.

The decision to treat a slow-growing tumor is often based on the type of symptoms that it causes, its location, and the amount of residual tumor present after surgery. For patients who have slow-growing tumors with very little residual disease, the risk of radiation therapy, chemotherapy, and other forms of treatment may outweigh the potential benefit, particularly if the patient does not have symptoms. Your doctor may recommend careful follow-up with MRI and regular neurological examinations.

14. Several genetic studies and tests were done on my tumor, a malignant glioma. Which, if any, are important in my treatment and prognosis?

Many genetic tests are commercially available, and although some tests can be done on only fresh tissue, the majority can be done on blocks and slides, months or years after surgery. Because of the many new therapies that target specific genes (see Question 56), testing for genes that currently do not have a therapy that modifies their function may nevertheless be important in the future. For example, the signaling pathways phospho-inositide-3 kinase/Akt and ras/mitogen-activated protein kinase are found in 88% of glioblastoma tumor specimens, and both have been shown to be associated with poorer survival. Currently, however, no effective therapy has emerged that targets these particular markers.

One of the more common markers studied in glioblastoma that has prognostic significance is the DNA repair enzyme O6-methylguanine-DNA methyltransferase (MGMT). The loss, or the blocking of, this enzyme makes an individual more susceptible to DNA damage and possible tumor development. Also, the loss of MGMT makes the tumor cell more susceptible to DNA damage from radiation therapy and many chemotherapy agents, including BCNU, Temodar, and Cytoxan. In this way, the methylation of MGMT, which blocks its normal repair function, can predict whether the tumor cells will survive treatment by radiation therapy and some types of chemotherapy. However, the cells that had the normal DNA repair enzyme were unlikely to be affected by these drugs. In studies of Temodar-treated glioblastoma patients comparing those who had tumors with the normal MGMT with those who had tumors with the methylated (silenced) MGMT, the survival was poorer in the normal MGMT group. Because of this, some studies have separated patients based on the normal versus methylated MGMT status; patients with high levels of MGMT may be good candidates for another kind of treatment that is not affected by MGMT.

The *p53* gene, located on the short arm of chromosome 17, is one of the best characterized tumor suppressor genes, the mutation of which can disrupt cell function and transform a normal cell to a malignant cell. *p53* is altered in a variety of tumor types and may play a role in the transformation of a normal cell to glioblastoma, although it has been found in low grades of glioma as well.

Other commercially available biomarkers that may predict treatment response include epidermal growth factor receptor (EGFR), vascular endothelial growth factor (VEGF), and platelet-derived growth factor (PDGF). **Figure 5** is a partial list of some of the molecular targets discovered in malignant glioma. These are important targets for the new therapies that are being developed (see Figure 24, Part Six).

Another genetic marker commonly used in the oligodendrogliomas is the evaluation of chromosomes 1p and 19q. Deletion of both of these chromosomes appears to be associated with an improved survival and increased sensitivity to chemotherapy; the presence of both intact chromosomes is associated with poorer survival, with the presence of one of the two associated with an intermediate prognosis.

Another genetic marker commonly used in the oligodendrogliomas is the evaluation of chromosomes 1p and 19q.

AKT	Histone Deacetylase	PKC β2
Angiopoietin Inhibitors	Hsp90 Inhibitors	PLK Inhibitors
Aurora Kinase Inhibitors	IGFR	Proteosome
Chk Kinase Inhibitors	Integrins	RAF kinase
EGFR	mTOR	Src
Farnesyltransferase	PDGF	TGF-β/TGF-β Receptor
HGF	PI3K	VEGF/VEGFR
Hif-1α	PKC	

Figure 5   Partial List of Molecular Targets-Malignant Glioma

How to Read Your Pathology Report

1 The hospital or laboratory that produces the report, usually where the surgery was performed.

2 Patient's name, hospital or medical record number, and date of birth.

3 The unique number assigned to this case; the reference number to locate slides in the future.

4 The surgeon submitting the specimen.

5 The impression of the surgeon before diagnosis, often the reason for the procedure.

6 The surgeon's notes on the origin of the specimen.

7 The final diagnosis, which may appear before or after the more detailed descriptions of the specimen.

8 Preliminary diagnosis by "frozen section" is sometimes helpful to guide the surgeon who must decide whether to attempt to remove more tumor.

9 The dimensions and appearance of the tissue received.

10 This is the description of the tumor cells themselves. Key phrases include the following:

   a. Infiltrating neoplasm: Tumor cells that blend into the normal brain without a clear separation.

   b. Oligodendroglial differentiation: Based on the descriptions preceding this phrase, the pathologist comments about the probable origin of the tumor. In this case, the evidence suggests that the tumor derived from oligodendrocytes, rather than astrocytes, ependymal cells, etc.

   c. Focal hemorrhage: Small collections of blood within the tumor.

   d. Necrosis: Literally means dead cells. Often, tumors that have a rapid rate of growth show these areas that have not had sufficient blood supply to allow continued growth.

   e. Heightened cellularity: The increased density of cells in a specific area, compared with what would normally be expected.

   f. Pleomorphism: Literally means many forms, depicting a variety of cell sizes and shapes.

   g. Vascular proliferation: An increase in the number of cells lining the walls of blood vessels of the tumor.

   h. Mitotic activity: The activity of cells that are dividing, often seen as dark, irregularly shaped nuclei.

   i. Anaplastic: Growing without structure or form; not resembling orderly normal tissue.

11 M1B-1 staining determines how many cells in a specimen are synthesizing DNA in preparation of cell division; it provides an estimate for the rate of tumor growth.

12 The pathologist who reviews the slides and determines the final diagnosis.

St. Mark's Medical Center 1 *
Fordham Ridge, Massachusetts

Doe, John Q. 2

MR No. 393898882

DOB: 6/26/52

Physician: John Smith, MD 4

Specimen No. S02-887999 3

Procedure Date: 7/25/09

Date of Report: 7/26/09

CLINICAL HISTORY: Right frontal brain tumor 5

DESCRIPTION OF SPECIMEN: Brain, right frontal mass 6

FINAL DIAGNOSIS: Anaplastic oligodendroglioma 7

INTRAOPERATIVE CONSULT: 8

An intraoperative consultation with frozen section is diagnosed as marked edema, favor low-grade glioma; defer final diagnosis to permanent sections. Conveyed to Dr. Smith 7/25/09 by Dr. Jones.

GROSS DESCRIPTION: 9

Specimen A is received fresh for frozen section labeled "right frontal brain mass" and consists of several soft, tan-gray irregular fragments of tissue that measure 0.8 × 0.4 × 0.3 cm in aggregate. The entire specimen is submitted. Specimen B is received fresh labeled "right frontal brain mass" and consists of a 3.5 × 3.8 × 2.2 cm soft, gray to gray-white wedge shaped portion of brain tissue. The entire specimen is submitted.

MICROSCOPIC DESCRIPTION: 10

Sections reveal an infiltrating neoplasm dominated by cells with generally rounded nuclei, variably developed perinuclear halos, microcystic change, and a delicate branching capillary network consistent, in aggregate, with oligodendroglial differentiation. There is focal hemorrhage present, but no frank necrosis is seen. Although much of the lesion appears low-grade, the neoplasm contains areas of heightened cellularity, pleomorphism, early vascular proliferation, and mitotic activity, with up to 2 mitotic figures per high power field, commensurate with an anaplastic (Grade III) lesion. Immunohistochemical stains reveal a moderate to high MIB-1 labeling index, with labeling of approximately 10% of the neoplastic cells in the more active areas, also commensurate with an anaplastic grade lesion. 11

Dr. Jones and Dr. Brown have reviewed the slides and agree with the final diagnosis.

Signed by: Jane Black, MD 12

Entered: 7/26/09 1530

*Names are fictional throughout

15. Will my brain tumor spread to another part of my body? Can it spread to another part of my brain or spinal cord?

Primary brain tumors that originate in the brain, such as gliomas, rarely metastasize, or spread, to other organs of the body. Some rare primary brain tumors that do metastasize include pituitary carcinoma, hemangioperi-cytoma, and papillary meningioma.

Primary or metastatic brain tumors may spread throughout the central nervous system (CNS) through the spinal fluid, sometimes causing symptoms such as back pain, weakness, or numbness. **Leptomeningeal metastases** (see Question 16) may be seen on an MRI as a coating around the brain or spinal cord. The MRI may also show tiny tumors, called "drop" metastases, in the lower spinal cord. Some common systemic cancers associated with leptomeningeal metastases include breast cancer, small cell lung cancer, lymphoma, and melanoma. Primary brain tumors that can spread throughout the spinal fluid include primary CNS lymphoma, germ cell tumors, glioblastoma, and medulloblastoma.

Some primary brain tumors have multiple sites in the brain at diagnosis and are termed **multifocal**. CNS lymphoma, germinomas, and less commonly malignant gliomas can appear at multiple sites in the brain. Biopsy of at least one area is necessary to distinguish between a multifocal primary tumor and a metastatic tumor because treatment recommendations for these tumor types may differ.

16. How are metastatic tumors different from primary brain tumors?

Good question! Although they may appear similar in initial symptoms and in their appearance on scans, metastatic tumors have an origin outside of the brain. The mass in the brain may cause symptoms before diagnosis of the tumor of origin, or primary tumor. Identification of the primary tumor is important because different kinds of tumors do not respond to the same treatment (i.e., breast, lung, kidney, and melanoma do not respond to the same medications and may respond differently to radiation therapy).

Sometimes a pathologist is able to identify the tumor clearly as metastatic (because of its appearance microscopically) despite a thorough and negative, search for its origin. Such tumors are called "metastatic tumors of unknown primary." These tumors are often more difficult to treat because a specific treatment plan cannot be recommended.

As noted in Question 4, metastatic tumors are much more common than primary brain tumors. Over 150,000 people with cancer are estimated to have brain metastases; some may develop metastatic disease to the brain years after their initial diagnosis. Although many metastatic tumors are discrete nodules or masses within the brain (Figures 6 and 7), some tumors develop as tiny nodules or sheets of cells covering the brain and spinal cord; such tumors are referred to as leptomeningeal metastases. Breast cancer is the most common tumor that spreads in this way, although lymphoma, melanoma, and lung cancer may also show **leptomeningeal spread**.

There is a complex interaction between tumor cells in the bloodstream and the blood vessels of the brain. Although some tumor cells may be destroyed by the immune system before they are able to form a tumor mass, it appears that some are able to adhere to the lining of the blood vessels of the brain (the endothelium)

Leptomeningeal spread

The spread of cancer cells through the spinal fluid, producing a coating around the brain or spinal cord.

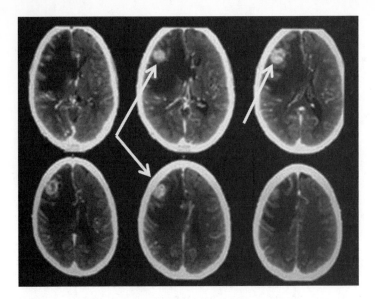

Figure 6   Lung tumors that spread though the bloodstream and to the brain may appear as multiple enhancing lesions.

Source: Reproduced from Dr. K. Hatantaa, M.D., Neuropathologist, University of Texas Southwestern Medical School, Dallas, TX.

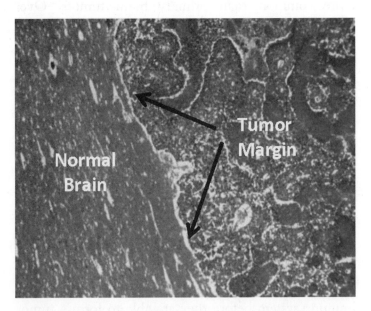

Figure 7   Adenocarcinoma of the lung invades the normal brain.

Source: Reproduced from Dr. K. Hatantaa, M.D., Neuropathologist, University of Texas Southwestern Medical School, Dallas, TX.

and invade the brain. A variety of substances, including neurotropins, plasmins, and matrix metalloproteinases, have been shown to stimulate brain invasion. In addition, small clusters of tumor cells produce VEGF, which promotes new blood vessel growth. This allows micrometastases to become larger, more destructive tumors but also explains why many brain metastases, while otherwise resembling their tissue of origin, are more vascular. It is well known, for example, that malignant melanoma in the brain is associated with a high risk of spontaneous hemorrhage.

A brain metastasis may be indistinguishable on MRI or CT from a primary brain tumor, particularly when a single lesion is present. Most metastatic tumors enhance with contrast, although some may appear solid and others cystic. A solitary brain metastasis may be treated surgically or with radiation therapy if the primary tumor is known. If the patient does not have a history of cancer or if a primary tumor cannot be identified, surgery may be necessary to identify the origin of the tumor.

Treatment recommendations for metastatic tumors are usually different from primary brain tumors; often the patient with metastatic cancer will have multiple other tumors throughout the body. For this reason, patients with metastatic brain tumors often have a less successful outcome than those with primary brain tumors.

PART THREE

Neuroimaging

I had a CT scan that was abnormal, but then the
doctor also ordered an MRI scan. Why do I need both?

How does an MRI work?

I have had surgery and radiation therapy
for a brain tumor. How often should I have a
follow-up MRI scan?

More . . .

17. I had a seizure at work and was brought to the emergency room. I had a CT scan that was abnormal, but then the doctor also ordered an MRI scan. Why do I need both?

Most patients have both a CT scan and an MRI because they provide different information.

Most patients have both a CT scan and an MRI because they provide different information. Many emergency rooms use CT (computed tomography) scans as an initial screen for tumors, stroke, hemorrhage, and other neurological conditions. CT is more widely available, less expensive, and can be done in a matter of minutes. MRI (magnetic resonance imaging) typically takes much longer and may not be immediately available. Some patients cannot have an MRI because they have metal pacemakers or other metal devices implanted in their bodies; however, an MRI does not use X-rays or iodine contrast, which makes it safer for most patients. In addition, an MRI provides more detailed, three-dimensional pictures of the brain. These detailed pictures are particularly important when planning surgery.

CT scans typically show only a single plane of the brain (an **axial image**). Axial images are slices through the brain that begin at the crown and end at the bottom of the skull. They are useful because right and left hemispheres of the brain are normally mirror images of each other. It is easy to see any distortion of one of the hemispheres with an axial image. Two other types of imaging planes, sagittal and coronal, are typically seen only with an MRI. A **sagittal image** divides the brain into left and right, as if divided from the tip of the nose to the center of the back of the head. This type of image is particularly helpful in showing tumors located in the exact center of the brain and its depth related to the skull. **Coronal images** divide the brain into front

Axial image

An image that begins at the crown and ends at the base of the skull, revealing the left and right halves of the brain.

Sagittal image

An image that divides the brain into left and right hemispheres and is particularly good at showing tumors in the exact center of the brain.

(anterior) and back (posterior), and they show the deeper and more central areas of the brain and whether there is any distortion of the midline structures. Each image on an MRI includes other information, such as the thickness of the slice in millimeters, the number in the sequence, and the right and left orientation of coronal and axial images (**Figure 8**).

Coronal image

Image that divides the brain into front (anterior) and back (posterior) and shows the best deeper and more central areas of the brain.

Neuroimaging

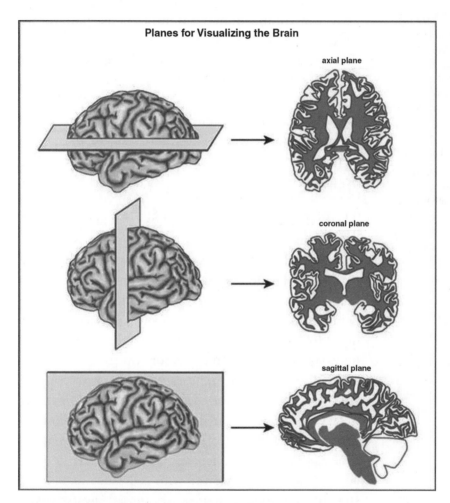

Planes for Visualizing the Brain

axial plane

coronal plane

sagittal plane

Figure 8 CT scans and MRI scans create images in "slices," which are reconstructed in three planes to give the exact dimension and location of tumors.

Source: Reproduced with permission from *Stahl's Essential Psychopharmacology,* Cambridge University Press, 2009.

Also, you may notice that an MRI series has many more images than a typical CT series. Several specific "sequences" are included in most MRI series of the brain; these are not available with CT. These images may be particularly useful in evaluating the blood flow to the normal brain and to the tumor and in evaluating excess water (edema) surrounding the tumor. A complete MRI series often includes one or more views after the administration of intravenous **gadolinium** contrast. Gadolinium contrast is useful in MRI because it causes a marked change in the **radiosignal** wherever there is a breakdown of the blood–brain barrier. Some tumors are associated with a breakdown of the blood–brain barrier so consistently that their appearance on gadolinium-enhanced MRI scans is an important key in their diagnosis (see "How to Read Your Own MRI Scans" on page 55).

Gadolinium

A silvery-white, malleable rare-earth metal that is often used in intravenous compounds that enhance contrast in MRIs and other imaging.

Radiosignal

In MRI, the image produced by resonance of hydrogen atoms in a magnetic field during and after a radiofrequency pulse.

The first scans that you have (those that are performed before surgery and before any medications are prescribed, including steroids) are very important. These scans may be needed to help determine your treatment, especially if surgery and radiation therapy are being considered. Although many imaging facilities now store MRIs and other radiographic images digitally, you can and should ask for copies of your MRI and CT scans. Some facilities will charge for copying your scans but may not charge for a copy as long as it is taken to one of your doctors. With each follow-up scan, you should ask for a copy to be made at the same time as the original. These copies can be taken to your appointments and reviewed with your doctors, but you should keep them in your possession afterward. Many imaging facilities now copy radiographic images onto CDs, but some still use film; ask your doctors which one they prefer. Because several scans can be copied onto a single CD, this is a very convenient way to keep a copy of your scans or mail them to another physician for review. The only disadvantage with CDs is the side-by-side comparison of two separate scans—this is possible with some programs but is more convenient with film.

As you continue your treatment, you will need to have MRI scans on a regular basis. Your physicians typically will refer you to one particular facility so that your scans will be of consistently high quality and will be interpreted by an experienced neuroradiologist. It is critical that the neuroradiologist has access to the previous scans; if you must change imaging facilities, be sure to take copies of your scans with you to allow the neuroradiologist to compare the older images to your new scan. It is helpful, if you plan to review your new scan with your physicians, that you bring the most recent previous scan for comparison.

18. How does an MRI work?

This is extremely difficult to explain in layman terms, but the very name, magnetic resonance imaging, is a brief description of the principle of MRI. Everyone is familiar with magnets and the fact that magnets have a north pole and a south pole. There is a magnetic field of the Earth, but the magnetic force of an MRI is at least 1,000 times stronger than the Earth's magnetic force. The nuclei of the hydrogen molecules of the brain are magnets and have a north pole and a south pole. In the magnetic field of an MRI unit, all of the north poles of the hydrogen nuclei of the brain align in one direction. The MRI unit sends a radiosignal to the nuclei, which causes them to flip 90 degrees. When the radiosignal switches off, the nuclei go back to their original position. As the nuclei change position, they emit an electromagnetic signal (resonance) that is captured on a computer. The computer determines exactly where the signal is coming from, and it is this localization that produces an image. The strength of the electromagnetic signal from abnormal tissue in the brain is different from the signal from the normal brain, producing a different shade of gray or different radiosignal. Most patients suspected of having a tumor will be given an intravenous injection of gadolinium. The gadolinium contrast agent defines certain areas of the brain that do not have an intact blood–brain barrier, such as the pituitary and pineal glands, as well as some tumors.

Although it is an oversimplification to say that an MRI detects the subtle differences in the hydrogen content of the structures of the brain, that is exactly what it does.

Although it is an oversimplification to say that an MRI detects the subtle differences in the hydrogen content of the structures of the brain, that is exactly what it does. All of the clicks, buzzes, and banging that you hear during an MRI examination are circuits causing the magnets of the hydrogen nuclei to flip back and forth. A typical MRI scan includes several different types of images. Each image provides different information and may be done in axial, coronal, or sagittal planes. Also, the thickness of the slices may be adjusted to allow better definition of small structures.

The most common MRI units use magnets with 1.5 Tesla; however, stronger magnets such as 3.0 Tesla are available in many centers. These units produce images with better resolution.

M.L.'s comment:

I have had a lot of MRI scans (well over a dozen now), and although I'm not claustrophobic, I can see why a lot of people would have a difficult time with an MRI. Lying on a table and having this machine slide you into what feels like a very cramped tunnel can make anyone feel like they need to get out! Some patients I know take a medication called Niravam, which is similar to the antianxiety drug Xanax, but works much faster. I haven't had to take anything, but I know it's important not to fidget. A technique that seems to work for me is to close my eyes and take deep breaths. I focus on the breath that I'm taking in and the one that I'm breathing out. I try not to think about the fact that I'm in a "tunnel." By using this technique, I usually come pretty close to falling asleep. Also, make sure that the MRI technician gives you some earplugs. The MRI machine can be kind of loud. The earplugs really help cut down on the noise, and sometimes they make it easier for me to fall asleep. When the technician gives me the contrast dye, I try not to let it get to me, but I just don't like being stuck with needles. Typically, technicians that insert IV catheters on a regular basis have the procedure down so well that they know how to do it so that it doesn't really hurt. I NEVER look at the location where the needle is being stuck; I just always make sure and tell the technician, "Please don't hurt me!" Even though my tumor hasn't shown any bright areas of contrast enhancement, I know that it's important to have the contrast anyway, because any change could be significant.

During the first year of my treatment, I had MRI scans every 3 months. When I completed treatment, I still had frequent MRI scans just to make sure that everything was stable, but in the last few years, I have gradually lengthened the time between scans. For a while, I was having scans every 6 months, but in July 2008, I had a series of seizures. Because my doctors wanted to make sure that there wasn't any tumor growth that had caused the seizures, I had to have more frequent MRI scans for the next several months. Although I know it's important to follow-up on any changes in my condition, my husband and I, especially my husband, breathe a little easier every time my MRI scan has come back "clean." The reason I say "especially my husband" is that I remember the best piece of advice that was given to me from a support group counselor: "If you cannot change the outcome of a situation then DO NOT worry about it." If you think about that statement, it makes a lot of sense, and it has really stuck with me over the years. I find myself practicing this in many areas of my life, especially when it's time for my next MRI scan. I know there isn't a thing I can do to change the outcome of that scan, so I do not worry about the results. If the results come back and they are not 100% positive, then I know there will be options for me to discuss with my neuro-oncologist. You might think that sounds a bit too simplistic, but if you find yourself worrying about MRI scan results or whether your tumor is going to come back, then I would encourage you to first think about what you can and cannot control. If you cannot change the outcome, then do not worry about it because worrying about something that you cannot change will only cause more stress and fear. If you focus your efforts on situations that you CAN control, such as your treatments and follow-up, then you will be directing your energy in a positive way and hopefully will find that your stress levels will decrease significantly.

19. I have had surgery and radiation therapy for a brain tumor. How often should I have a follow-up MRI scan?

Your doctor considers many factors when determining the frequency of follow-up MRI scans. Although there are no specific guidelines for the follow-up of brain tumors, a general rule is that if the result of the scan would have an impact on the patient's decision for further therapy, a scan is recommended.

For patients who have benign or very slow-growing tumors, such as meningiomas, scans may be required once a year or even less often, *if the patient is not having symptoms.* If the patient has developed headaches, for example, and has a meningioma that has been stable for several years, it is possible that the headaches are entirely unrelated; however, both doctor and patient are reassured if a follow-up scan shows no new abnormalities.

On the other hand, more aggressive tumors, such as a glioblastoma or a primary central nervous system (CNS) lymphoma, may show evidence of growth even when MRI scans are taken 1 month apart. For patients who are undergoing treatment such as radiation therapy or chemotherapy, oncologists usually recommend a follow-up scan at the end of the treatment cycle, which may be 4 weeks, 6 weeks, or even longer, depending on the treatment. Patients who are being treated on a clinical trial are required to have scans at specific points in time designated by the treatment protocol. In the absence of any new symptoms, oncologists will usually recommend evaluation of the response to treatment just before a new cycle begins.

Upon completion of treatment, most patients continue to have scans at regular intervals—longer intervals for slower growing tumors and shorter intervals for aggressive tumors. Follow-up scans may detect very small tumors before they cause symptoms. In some cases, these smaller tumors are amenable to specific kinds of treatments, such as **Gamma Knife** radiosurgery, that would be impossible if the tumor was larger.

Patients with metastatic tumors typically have to be reevaluated for all of the sites of their disease after

Gamma Knife
Type of stereotactic radiation designed to deliver radiation from multiple cobalt sources, computer-focused to a small area or multiple small areas.

Patients with metastatic tumors typically have to be reevaluated for all of the sites of their disease after treatment has been completed.

Neuroimaging

treatment has been completed. Some patients require CT scans of the chest and abdomen to evaluate the primary tumor. It may be more convenient for such patients to have a CT scan of the brain at the same time; however, if there is an area that is suspicious for a new tumor on the CT scan, an MRI may still be helpful because of its higher resolution. Again, the goal of imaging is to evaluate the success of previous treatment and to determine whether a new or residual tumor requires a change in treatment.

Patients often wonder whether there is some type of long-term injury from too many MRI scans. Recently, radiologists have become more aware of the side effects of the contrast agents used in both CT and MRI scans. Although we know of no definite injury from the magnetic resonance used in an MRI, MRI contrast (gadolinium) has caused allergic reactions and kidney damage.

Neuroradiologist

Physician trained to interpret X-rays, CT scans, and other radiological images of the brain.

How to Read
Your Own MRI Scans

Patients who have been diagnosed with a brain or spinal cord tumor are usually carrying around a huge X-ray file folder of their films to their neurosurgeon, radiation oncologist, or neuro-oncologist for months before they figure out that these films are, literally, the key to their future. A neuroradiologist can look at someone's brain MRI and predict what will happen next if the tumor continues to grow. For example, a neuroradiologist can tell if the patient's right leg will become weaker, if part of the patient's visual field will be lost, and if the patient will develop speech problems. Of course, most neuroradiologists do not actually see the patient. It is up to the doctor taking care of the patient to use the information provided by neuroradiologist to design an appropriate treatment strategy.

Neuroradiologists are doctors who have been trained in general radiology (interpreting a variety of images) and receive further training in the interpretation of images of the brain and spine. Neuroradiologists typically see thousands of brain tumor cases during their training. This experience gives them a unique advantage over most other radiologists and even other neurological specialists; however, learning some of the basic principles of MRI interpretation can be helpful to the patient (and almost every brain tumor patient has sneaked a peek at the new scans when given the opportunity).

If an MRI of your brain has already been done at another facility, bring it with you when you have a new scan, even if it is several months old. A neuroradiologist looks for *changes over time*. If your doctor is ordering an MRI scan now, even though you had one

3 months ago, it is because she is expecting that there are or could be changes in the appearance of the brain during the interval.

Second, a neuroradiologist looks for *changes in symmetry* (**Figure a**). The tumor or swelling around the tumor may have created a distortion of the center line of the brain called *midline shift* (**Figure b**). If the distortion involves compression against another section of the brain, this is called *mass effect*.

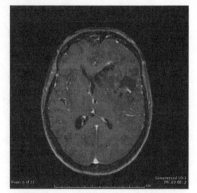

Figure a

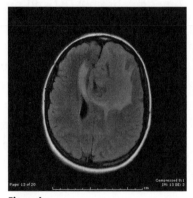

Figure b

Third, you have noticed that MRI scans are black and white images, and their interpretation depends on what can be subtle changes in gray scale, reflecting changes in the radiosignal. Black and white photographs have negatives, but MRI scans are not positive and negative images in the same sense. Although there are often several different kinds of images, or *sequences*, included in a complete MRI study of the brain, the T2-weighted (or T2 scans) and T1-weighted gadolinium-enhanced images (often marked with adhesive labels on film, or "post" on digital images) are among the most important.

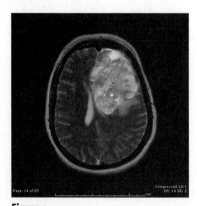

Figure c

Figure c is a T2-weighted axial image. This type of image shows the spinal fluid and any excess water in the brain as white.

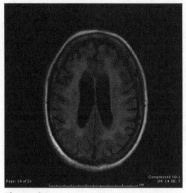

Figure d

Edema (swelling) around a tumor may be very striking, as in the image here. Another type of image, the FLAIR (**Figure d**), also shows edema well, but note that the water within the ventricles is not bright, as it is on the T2. Remember that your symptoms can be caused by this edema, which is why your doctor usually studies these images carefully.

Even when the tumor has been completely removed, there may still be a lighter margin around the area of the surgery for several months because T2 and FLAIR scans are so sensitive to residual water. Some types of tumors, including some low-grade gliomas, are detected only on T2 and FLAIR scans. Effects of radiation therapy can also show changes on these scans. Many other changes within the brain, including strokes, multiple sclerosis, and infection, can also cause changes on T2 and FLAIR scans. In addition, increased intracranial pressure, which forces spinal fluid into the surrounding white matter, is easily detected on FLAIR.

Figure e is an axial image of a primary CNS lymphoma after an intravenous injection of gadolinium contrast. The tumor is much more obvious with contrast because it has caused what neuroradiologists refer to as "breakdown of the blood–brain barrier." In other words, the presence of the tumor has created tiny leaks in the very fine blood vessel networks in the tumor. Other abnormalities of the brain can also show bright areas after the administration of contrast, including the changes that occur at the margin of the

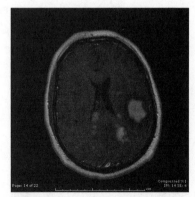

Figure e

Neuroimaging

tumor after surgery. For this reason, many neurosurgeons feel that MRIs can be misleading in judging how much tumor remains after surgery.

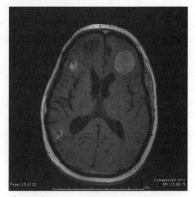

Figure f

Recent bleeding within the brain appears bright white before the administration of contrast. Because some tumors bleed spontaneously, it is important to compare the T1 images before and after the administration of contrast (**Figures f** and **g**).

One of the most difficult changes that a neuroradiologist must detect includes changes that occur as a result of therapy. A neuroradiologist usually does not know what therapy has been given. For example, a dense, white area on the scan of a patient who has received Gamma Knife or radiosurgery may be a recurrent, growing tumor or

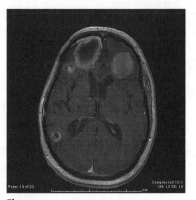

Figure g

may be dead tumor (radiation necrosis). It can be impossible to tell the difference (**Figure h**), and close follow-up may be required to determine whether the suspicious area is stable. In this case, the follow-up scans several months later show that the enhancing area has resolved, suggesting that the

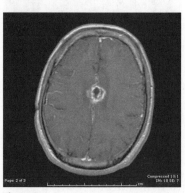

Figure h

abnormality was likely radiation induced (**Figure i**).

Figure j is the contrast-enhanced image of a patient who has a malignant glioma that was diagnosed 2 years before this scan was performed. The tumor causes a distortion of the normal structures of the brain, with both prominent mass effect on the lateral ventricle and midline shift from right to left. After the administration of gadolinium contrast, there is markedly increased radiosignal within the tumor. Although the tumor originated in the right frontal lobe, it has now crossed the corpus callosum and extends into the left frontal lobe.

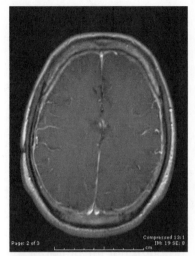

Figure i

Figure k is the T1-weighted, contrast-enhanced view that demonstrates multiple abnormalities distributed throughout several

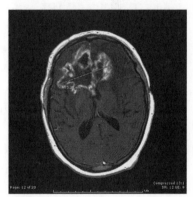

Figure j

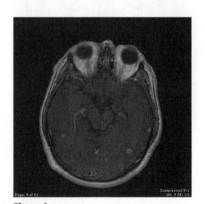

Figure k

lobes of the brain. In this patient with a known history of lung cancer, the abnormalities depicted are most consistent with metastatic lung cancer. Virtually all metastatic tumors enhance with contrast.

Figure l is a diffusion-weighted axial image showing multiple small

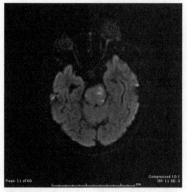

Figure l

bright areas in the brainstem. In this patient, who had previously received radiation near the brainstem, these bright abnormalities indicate recent vascular infarcts, or strokes. Typically, radiation-induced infarcts affect small vessels but can still be devastating, particularly in critical areas such as the brainstem.

Finally, it is unfortunate, although not uncommon, that tumors that have been changing slowly, if at all, on MRI scans may rapidly recur, even over a few weeks. **Figure m** is a T1-weighted, contrast-enhanced coronal view of a patient who has undergone previous surgery for an oligodendroglioma of the right frontal lobe. Eight weeks later, the same area shows that the tumor has recurred as a more aggressive, high-grade glioma (**Figure n**). Remember that even relatively subtle changes on an MRI may indicate that a change in therapy is indicated, and these changes may be detected only by performing MRI scans at regular intervals.

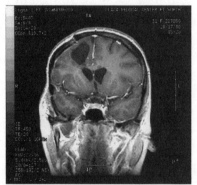

Figure m

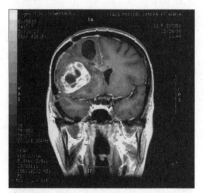

Figure n

20. After my surgery 2 years ago, I have had MRI scans regularly that have been stable. My most recent scan shows a new abnormality near the location of the original tumor. What are the chances that this is a new tumor? How can I find out?

Not every "new" area on an MRI scan of a brain tumor patient is a recurrence of the tumor—although the possibility of recurrence must be taken seriously. Some other abnormalities that may appear on an MRI scan include radiation treatment effects, vascular abnormalities, including stroke and "artifacts." Artifacts are false images that may be produced by the imaging process or by the movement of the patient. The neuroradiologist interpreting the scan compares all of the images in the series, including the coronal, axial, and sagittal sequences, to determine whether the "new" area is an artifact; however, it is not always possible to tell whether the new area appearing on the MRI is clearly related to the original tumor, particularly with a small abnormality.

Reviewing the scans with your physician may be helpful. He may recommend a follow-up MRI within 4 to 6 weeks to determine whether the abnormality is stable. Although a biopsy could be performed to determine whether the area seen on the MRI is a tumor, this would obviously involve more risk. Some abnormalities remain stable or even resolve completely over a period of a few weeks.

Not every "new" area on an MRI scan of a brain tumor patient is a recurrence of the tumor—although the possibility of recurrence must be taken seriously.

Neuroimaging

How to Read an MRI Report

1 Identification of the patient, the imaging facility, and the date of the scan.

2 Description of the study.

3 Diagnosis, or reason why the scan was ordered.

4 Description of the equipment used; in this case, the strength of the magnet.

5 List of the sequences included, including the imaging planes, the type and amount of contrast, and slice thickness.

6 Previous scans available for comparison.

7 Neuroradiologist's description of the scan. The neuroradiologist describes the abnormalities in relationship to the site of the original tumor. He describes the location of abnormalities (parasagittal = adjacent to the midline) and the changes since the previous scan ("progressive enlargement"). He measures the size of the enhancing lesions in millimeters, as seen on the T1 gadolinium-enhanced axial scan (the T2 or FLAIR abnormalities corresponding to these lesions is more difficult to measure precisely). A small lesion in the left frontal lobe is also identified. The neuroradiologist notes that there is no change in "perfusion" because rapidly growing tumors sometimes show an increase in blood flow or perfusion. Also, he notes that the lesions are "high signal" or bright on diffusion-weighted images, which may also reflect blood flow in high-grade tumors. In comparing all of these different sequences, the neuroradiologist affirms that the changes seen are consistent with tumor and not another process such as stroke or hemorrhage. The neuroradiologist comments on the stable abnormalities related to the previous craniotomy and tumor resection. He uses the term "encephalomalacia" (which literally means "brain softening") to describe the tissue around the resection site that has less blood flow as a result of surgery and radiation therapy.

8 Summary of the neuroradiologist's conclusions.

9 Neuroradiologist's name and medical degree.

10 Date and time of dictation.

Central Imaging of Alpharetta, GA 1
Date: July 30, 2010

PATIENT: PAULA ROPER; D.O.B. 5/7/54

MAGNETIC RESONANCE IMAGING OF THE BRAIN WITH AND WITHOUT 2
CONTRAST

CLINICAL INFORMATION: GLIOBLASTOMA 3

TECHNIQUE:

1. Images acquired with a **3-Tesla** magnetic resonance imaging device. 4
2. Sagittal 3-mm paramidline noncontrast T1-weighted images.
3. **Axial 3-mm T2, FLAIR, diffusion, perfusion and precontrast T1 images,** C1 to vertex. 5
4. Following **intravenous infusion of 20 cc of OptiMARK**, axial and coronal 3-mm thick T1-weighted images thorough the brain.

COMPARISON: Comparison is made to multiple previous examinations, the most recent of which is dated June 17, 2010. 6

FINDINGS: There is an irregular centrally cavitary **peripherally enhancing lesion** 7 in the **parasagittal** right frontal lobe, superior to the original tumor bed. This has demonstrated subtle but progressive enlargement over the series of examinations since March 18, 2008. The lesion is approximately 8 x 14 mm in greatest dimension. There is a small enhancing lesion in the **subcortical** white matter of the parasagittal left frontal lobe. This lesion is also slightly larger than the one present on the study of June 17, 2008. No definite change in the **perfusion images** is noted; however, this is a small lesion and at the limits of resolution for characterization by perfusion imaging. As noted before, these lesions are high signal on the **diffusion-weighted** images.

There is right frontal craniotomy with the bone flap in good position.
There is postsurgical **encephalomalacia** to the right frontal lobe, reflecting previous tumor resection.

There is no **hydrocephalus**.

IMPRESSION: 8

There are foci of cavitary enhancement in the high right frontal lobe, which have increased progressively over the studies from March 18, 2008.

There is a small enhancing lesion in the subcortical left frontal lobe, also larger than on the most recent study.

In view of the progressive enlargement, it is not possible to exclude the presence of recurrent tumor at these locations.

Joel Buschman, M.D. Board Certified Neuro-Radiology 9
Dictated: July 30, 2010; 2:32 p.m. 10

Figure 9   MRI report and images corresponding to the report. Each of these axial images is at the same area of the brain, but depicts the abnormality in a different way. Radiologists use the entire series to help distinguish tumor from stroke, scar tissue, etc.

These are the 6 Axial Sequences that the Neuroradiologist Uses in his Interpretations

Diffusion Weighted Imaging (DWI).

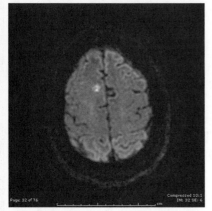

Perfusion.

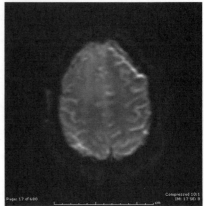

T2.

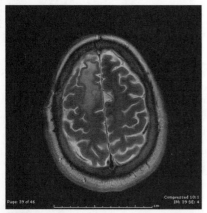

T1.

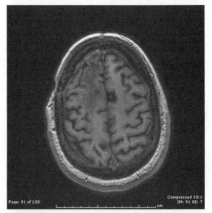

FLAIR.

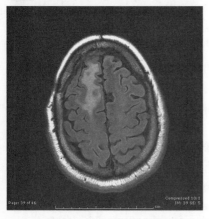

Gadolinium.

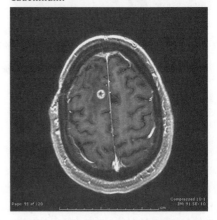

21. What is a PET scan? Should I have one? Why does my doctor use MRI scans and not PET scans to evaluate my tumor?

Positron emission tomography (PET) is an important imaging tool for many types of cancer and many types of CNS disease (Color Plate 3). Whereas CT and MRI scans reveal the structure (anatomy) of the body, PET scans reveal the differences in living tissues (physiology). PET scans require the administration of a radioactive substance, often a radioactive sugar, such as fluoro-deoxy-glucose (FDG), produced in a cyclotron. Several radioactive elements can be used in PET scanning, and they all have an atomic nucleus that undergoes transformation from a proton (a positively charged subatomic particle) into a neutron (a neutral subatomic particle). As a result of this transformation, a positron is released. The positron then combines with an electron, which produces energy in the form of gamma rays. The PET scanner detects the energy formed from the gamma rays, which is then reconstructed to form an image. PET images do not have the fine detail of MRI scans, but they do show differences in the **metabolism**, or use of energy, by the brain's cells.

More than 50 years ago, scientists discovered that glucose is taken up by living cells and that rapidly growing cancer cells take up more glucose than normal cells. Although early studies using PET suggested that the radioactive tracer FDG correlates with the rapid reproduction of cancer cells, more recent studies suggest that there is a correlation between the number of living cancer cells present. However, other conditions, such as infection, may also take up radioactive glucose at higher rates than normal tissue. Thus, high FDG uptake does not necessarily indicate cancer.

Positron emission tomography (PET)
A nuclear medicine imaging test that detects differences in metabolism; often used to differentiate between healthy and abnormal tissue.

Metabolism
The normal physical and chemical changes within living tissue.

Neuroimaging

The difference in uptake of FDG in normal brain tissue and in slower-growing tumors may be slight; therefore, PET has been used to differentiate between malignant or aggressive tumors (which show more intensely in the scan, indicating more radioactive tracer in this area) and more slow-growing tumors (which can show about the same amount of radioactive tracer as the normal brain). Before treatment, higher rates of FDG uptake in brain tumors have been shown in some studies to be associated with a poorer prognosis. After radiation treatment, FDG-PET can be used to distinguish between a residual living tumor and a tumor that is dead but still shows contrast enhancement on an MRI or a CT scan.

Some limitations exist, however, in using PET to monitor the patient's response to brain tumor therapy. After therapy, many patients have both tumor **necrosis** and residual, living tumor present in the brain. A PET scan that shows high FDG uptake suggests that there is living tumor present, but a low FDG uptake does not mean that the brain is tumor-free. Small amounts of living tumor could be present.

Necrosis

The premature, localized death of cells and living tissue.

Total body PET scans are frequently used in the evaluation of patients with lung cancer, breast cancer, and melanoma to detect metastases in the bones, lungs, liver, and other organs. Although larger brain metastases may also be detected in these total-body scans, small metastases may be missed, and an MRI of the brain may be necessary for this reason. In general, a tumor that is smaller than 1 centimeter (0.5 inch) may not be visible with a PET.

Finally, because a PET requires the administration of a radioisotope, many physicians limit patients to three or four studies per year. A negative pregnancy test is also required for women of child-bearing potential.

22. What is magnetic resonance spectroscopy? What does it tell my doctor about my tumor that the MRI does not?

Magnetic resonance spectroscopy (MRS) is a technique that is similar to conventional MRI that measures chemical compounds within the brain. Although conventional MRI detects differences in brain water, MRS techniques suppress brain water so that other compounds such as choline, creatine, and N-acetyl aspartate (NAA) can be detected. Detecting these compounds produces a chemical waveform or spectra in a tumor that can be compared with the spectra of an area of normal brain in the same patient. The amount of each of these compounds present in an area of the brain that appears abnormal on conventional MRI can suggest not only the presence of a tumor, but also the grade of tumor and whether necrosis is present. For example, because NAA is associated with living, normal neurons, a reduction in the NAA peak reflects an absence of neurons. On the other hand, the choline peak on an MRS is typically higher in brain tumors than in a normal brain because choline is associated with cell membrane metabolism and dense, rapidly proliferating tumors. Creatine, the third compound, may be either lower or higher than the choline peak in a brain tumor. Areas of necrosis may reveal a fourth peak on an MRS that corresponds to lactate.

The waveform or spectra from the normal brain and from the tumor are compared to reveal the proportion of NAA, creatine, and choline present in the tissue.

Magnetic resonance spectroscopy (MRS) is a technique that is similar to conventional MRI that measures chemical compounds within the brain.

Magnetic resonance spectroscopy (MRS)

A study similar to conventional MRI that measures chemical compounds within the brain.

Neuroimaging

These proportions are clearly different for the two areas, and radiologists who interpret MRS use this information to detect whether the abnormal areas are more likely to be tumor or necrosis (dead or dying cells). The changes in the spectra can also be evaluated after therapy to determine whether a viable tumor remains.

MRS has some advantages over PET in that it uses available MRI technology and does not require the use of contrast or radioisotopes. It can be repeated a number of times without risk to the patient; however, MRS has some limitations. MRS may be difficult to interpret in areas of the brain adjacent to the skull. The resolution of an MRS scan is relatively poor, making it unsuitable for the detection of small abnormalities. Like other imaging modalities, MRS cannot reliably differentiate between different tumor types and grades, although future developments in MRS may increase its accuracy.

23. After radiation therapy and initial chemotherapy, I was surprised to see that my tumor actually looked larger than it did before treatment. I wasn't having any new symptoms, but my oncologist said one of two things might be happening: growth of the tumor despite my treatment or something called "pseudoprogression." What is pseudoprogression?

Although an MRI is an excellent way to follow the course of a tumor, an MRI can be still limited in the ability to distinguish between living cells (tumor growth) and dead cells (necrosis). Both living and dead tumor cells can show bright areas with gadolinium contrast, and both can result in an apparent increase in the size of

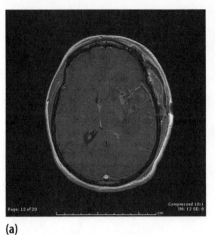

(a)

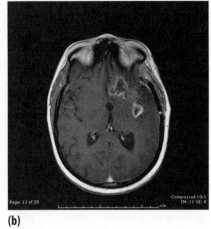

(b)

Figure 10   Pseudoprogression: (a) postop; (b) postradiation. The apparent increase in size and the well-defined enhancing areas can appear to be growth of the tumor after treatment. See Figure 11, over time, the size and enhancement decrease as the same therapy is continued. This suggests pseudoprogression.

the tumor (**Figure 10**). The neurological symptoms (or lack thereof) may not clearly show any correlation with the MRI findings in such cases.

Pseudoprogression is always limited to the original tumor area and radiation treatment field. Because it represents an area of dead or dying tumor, its presence need not cause concern that the patient must abandon the planned course of therapy. In other words, as the success of therapy actually produced the appearance on MRI, treatment should continue, with follow-up MRI scans often showing improvement within a few months (**Figure 11**).

There are several ways to determine whether the area seen on an MRI scan represents "true progression" or "pseudoprogression." Both FDG-PET and MRS (see Questions 21 and 22) may be helpful in showing metabolic changes characteristic of dead tissue. Also, a biopsy or resection of the suspicious area may be warranted, particularly if the patient's condition is deteriorating.

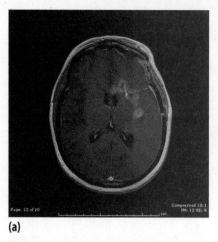 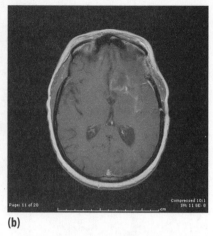

(a)   (b)

Figure 11   Pseudoprogression: (a) 1 month postradiation; (b) 2 months postradiation. With continued treatment, the enhancement and size of the tumor gradually improve.

However, even surgical removal does not always reveal whether the area on MRI was pseudoprogression or true progression, as the removed tissue may contain a mixture of living and dead tissue.

It is important to continue the planned course of therapy if pseudoprogression is likely. Some other treatments, however, have been studied to reduce the edema associated with pseudoprogression. These include steroids, hyperbaric oxygen, and recently, a new drug, Avastin.

24. I have read that functional MRI can show the parts of the brain that control movement and speech. Do I need a functional MRI before my surgery?

Functional MRI

A type of MRI that detects the changes in red blood cells and capillaries as they deliver oxygen to "functioning" parts of the brain.

Functional MRI, like conventional MRI imaging, detects differences in the magnetic properties of brain tissue, blood vessels, and spinal fluid. In addition, a functional MRI detects changes in red blood cells and capillaries as they deliver oxygen to "functioning" parts of the brain. For example, although it would be easy to assume that the entire brain is involved in complex activities such as speech, there are, in fact, very discrete areas of the brain that produce spoken language. These areas actually have higher blood flow and higher oxygen consumption when a person speaks. Functional MRI can detect these subtle but definite differences in oxygen consumption. A map of some of the functions of the brain can be developed by asking the patient to perform specific tasks, such as finger tapping, reading silently, or looking at pictures during an MRI (Color Plate 4).

Obviously, some of the more interesting, unique talents that people have, such as artistic or musical ability, are impossible to map with functional MRI.

Functional MRI for localizing certain brain areas before surgery may be useful. For example, a left-handed patient may have a tumor in the left frontal lobe that seems to extend into the area involved in the production of speech. Language dominance in most right-handed individuals is centered in the left hemisphere, but in some left-handed patients, language dominance is in the right hemisphere. Functional MRI can quickly and accurately determine the area of the brain involved in speech when the patient silently performs a series of word-recognition tasks. This may guide the neurosurgeon around the area (if the speech area localizes on the left near the tumor) or may give him reassurance that he will avoid it completely (if it localizes to the right hemisphere, opposite the tumor).

Functional MRI is not yet widely available, and relatively few situations require preoperative assessment with it. If your neurosurgeon believes that a functional MRI may be helpful in planning your surgery, he may discuss this with you.

PART FOUR

Neurosurgery

Is surgery necessary to diagnose a brain tumor?

What are the potential complications of a
neurosurgical procedure?

Should I get a second opinion before having
an operation?

More . . .

25. Is surgery necessary to diagnose a brain tumor?

Although a brain scan can show an abnormality that looks like a tumor, the only way to determine whether the abnormality is a tumor is by examination of a sample of the abnormality under the microscope.

Neurosurgeon

Surgeon specializing in the diagnosis and treatment of disease of the central and peripheral nervous systems, including the skull, spine, and blood vessels.

Resection

Surgical removal of a tumor; see also gross total resection and partial resection.

Although a brain scan can show an abnormality that looks like a tumor, the only way to determine whether the abnormality is a tumor is by examination of a sample of the abnormality under the microscope. Although there are many ways to obtain a sample of a suspected tumor, with rare exceptions, all of them involve some type of surgery.

Surgeons who operate on the brain and spinal cord have several years of specific training and are called **neurosurgeons**. A neurosurgeon interviews the patient, examines the medical records and scans, and then discusses with the patient the approach to determining the diagnosis. A neurosurgeon usually recommends one of two approaches: a biopsy or a **resection**.

A biopsy is the removal of a piece of the tumor that will be examined by a pathologist. An **open biopsy** involves removing a small amount of the tumor by carefully cutting through the scalp, skull, meninges, and the brain over the tumor. A **stereotactic biopsy** is the removal of a small piece of the tumor using computer guidance. Often the procedure involves placing a thin needle through a tiny opening in the scalp and skull. The neurosurgeon will decide which of these procedures is the most appropriate for the patient, depending on many factors.

Some patients have tumors that can be completely removed in a procedure called **gross total resection**. If only part of the tumor can be removed because of its size or location, the neurosurgeon may perform a **partial resection**. Removal of all or part of the tumor provides enough cells for the pathologist to examine under the microscope. When neurosurgeons describe a tumor that can be safely removed, they refer to it as **resectable**.

An open biopsy or resection that removes a part of the skull is called a **craniotomy**. In most cases, the opening in the skull is replaced with the section of bone that was removed to obtain the sample of the tumor. In a few cases, metal mesh or another type of material is placed over the brain if the bone must be removed permanently.

A few instances do not allow the examination of a piece of the tumor to confirm the diagnosis. Tumors in the brainstem or spinal cord may be difficult to biopsy because of the risk of damage to the blood vessels or normal structures nearby. Metastatic brain tumors that have spread from another cancer, such as a lung cancer or kidney cancer, may be removed if the neurosurgeon determines that the patient will benefit from their removal. Not all metastatic tumors require biopsy to confirm the diagnosis if the patient has already had a biopsy that determined the origin of the tumor. Finally, a few tumors, such as a germinoma or a primary central nervous system (CNS) lymphoma, may be diagnosed without surgery if tumor cells are present in the spinal fluid. Such patients may have a sampling of spinal fluid taken during a **spinal tap** or **lumbar puncture**. In all cases, a biopsy is needed to confirm diagnosis so that an appropriate treatment can be determined.

Sometimes tumors are found that appear to grow very slowly and have few, if any, symptoms. In these cases, a biopsy can be delayed for months or years. In the unusual circumstance that the patient is too ill to have any form of treatment, a biopsy may not be recommended.

Neurosurgery

Open biopsy

Procedure allowing a neurosurgeon to directly visualize the surface of the brain prior to the removal of a piece of a tumor.

Stereotactic biopsy

Removal of a small piece of the tumor using computer guidance, often with a thin needle placed through a tiny opening in the scalp and skull.

Gross total resection

Removal of all visible portions of a tumor.

Partial resection

Procedure that allows a neurosurgeon to directly visualize the surface of the brain prior to the removal of some, but not all, of a tumor.

Resectable

Able to be surgically removed.

Craniotomy

A surgical "cutting" of an opening into the skull.

Spinal tap

See lumbar puncture.

Lumbar puncture

Method of obtaining a sampling of spinal fluid from the space between the lumbar vertebrae.

The neurosurgeon is trained to make an appropriate evaluation of the patient's circumstances and will recommend surgery only if absolutely necessary.

26. What are the potential complications of a neurosurgical procedure?

The neurosurgeon will discuss with you the potential complications of the procedure that he recommends. Although a biopsy may remove a smaller piece of the tumor than a gross total resection, either procedure can be technically difficult depending on the size and location of the tumor. Like all surgical procedures, the possibility of bleeding, infection, and pain will be discussed with you. In many cases, the risks of the procedure can be minimized with careful planning and preparation.

Nondiagnostic

A tissue sample that does not contain adequate information for determining the presence or absence of disease.

For stereotactic or needle biopsies, which remove only a tiny piece of the tumor, the pathologist may determine that the biopsy is **nondiagnostic**. This means that no definite conclusions can be made about the tumor after careful review. In some cases, the small piece of tissue is crushed and the cells are distorted. In other cases, the tumor cells are adjacent to normal cells, and the biopsy needle removes only a sampling of normal cells. There is a higher risk of a nondiagnostic biopsy if the sample removed is very small. If a diagnosis cannot be determined, no treatment can be recommended, and therefore, another biopsy must be done. This is extremely frustrating for the pathologist, the neurosurgeon, and most of all, the patient.

More extensive neurosurgical procedures, such as partial and complete resections, may be needed to provide a sample of the tumor to the pathologist as well as relieve pressure caused by the tumor. The difficulty of removing a tumor and the possible risks of removing it depend on multiple factors, including the size and location of the tumor, the blood vessels in and around the tumor, and any previous surgery or radiation therapy performed on the same area. Some patients in poor health may have heart or lung problems that would prolong recovery from surgery. Although neurological functions such as motor strength or coordination may become impaired immediately after surgery, in many cases, these deficits resolve with time and rehabilitation. The risk of seizure after a neurosurgical procedure is low in most patients; however, many neurosurgeons use antiseizure medication (anticonvulsants) routinely in the postoperative setting.

27. I was taken to my local emergency room and told that I have a brain tumor. The neurosurgeon on call told me that I would need surgery right away. Should I get a second opinion before having an operation?

Second opinions can be a good idea. Almost everyone who has to make a serious decision wants to consider all of the options carefully. No one wants to feel rushed into a decision about surgery, but some tumors cause life-threatening symptoms or grow so quickly that surgery should be done as soon as possible. As the patient, you need to know whether you have a few days to consider your options or to seek an opinion from another neurosurgeon.

A neurosurgeon should be able to explain in detail the operation that he is planning and what he expects to find. Although some tumor types are difficult to predict based on the appearance of the scans, a neurosurgeon should be able to explain why he expects a primary or metastatic tumor and whether it is benign or malignant (although only the pathologist can say for certain; that is why the surgery is necessary!). He should be honest about the equipment and the hospital and whether he has access to the most up-to-date technology. The neurosurgeon should also be well versed in options such as genetic or chemosensitivity assays if they are required for the type of tumor that you have. Although he may not be able to answer every question that you (or your family) may have, the neurosurgeon should never appear to be dismissive or uninformed. There are, after all, neurosurgeons all over the country who are well trained in the treatment of brain tumors; other neurosurgeons are also good surgeons, but they may specialize in the complexity of spinal surgery, vascular surgery, or peripheral nerve surgery. Obviously, you will want to know that the neurosurgeon assigned to you from the emergency room is experienced in the treatment of brain tumors.

Neurosurgeons, like most other specialists, are trained over several years and are only then allowed to take board certification examinations. Your neurosurgeon should be board certified in neurosurgery. You can find this out by checking: www.abns.org/diplomates.

If you have reservations about the neurosurgeon after your initial consultation, you should speak frankly to your neurosurgeon about your concerns. Tell him that you are considering a second opinion because of the seriousness of the surgery. Ask, "If you had to have this operation, who would you select as your neurosurgeon and why?" His answer should reflect his knowledge of neurosurgeons who operate on brain tumors frequently and who have a reputation for excellent patient care. Asking this question is not insulting; after all, you are indicating that you trust his judgment.

M.L.'s comment:

Regarding a second opinion, my answer would be this: it depends. You may not need one, or you may not have time to get one. If you've had a seizure and your doctor thinks that you may have a fast-growing tumor, you may not have several days to obtain a second opinion. If speaking to another doctor makes you feel more comfortable, however, then you should do so. These days, getting a second opinion is a fairly common practice. In some cases, your insurance company may even require it, especially if surgery is recommended. The most important thing to remember is that you must be sure that it's safe for you to delay your treatment long enough to obtain a second opinion. I was extremely fortunate to have an excellent neurosurgeon. He referred me to other doctors who were also excellent in providing my follow-up care.

28. Are there some brain tumors that can be surgically cured? Is a tumor that cannot be resected always incurable?

Some brain tumors are surgically cured; one of the most common tumors, meningioma, can be completely resected and cured. A number of other tumors, including acoustic neuroma, central neurocytoma, subependymoma, and dysembryoplastic neuroepithelial tumor, to name a few, may not recur after complete resection. Some tumors, even if not completely resected, grow back so slowly that another operation may not be needed for many years. Tumors that are completely resected and do not tend to grow back are considered benign; however, benign tumors in certain locations in the brain may still cause death if they cannot be safely removed.

Some tumors cannot be resected surgically; nevertheless, if they respond to other forms of treatment such as radiation therapy or chemotherapy, complete surgical

Some brain tumors are surgically cured; one of the most common tumors, meningioma, can be completely resected and cured.

resection may not be necessary. Germinomas, lymphomas, and other tumors that commonly occur in the deep structures of the brain are often difficult to resect. Fortunately, many can be treated successfully with chemotherapy, radiation therapy, or both.

29. I have seen two neurosurgeons about surgery for my brain tumor, and both say that my tumor can be safely removed. One of them says that he uses "MRI guidance" to remove the tumor. What does this mean? Is there an advantage to using MRI to remove the tumor?

Neuronavigation

Preoperative or intraoperative imaging information that allows the surgeon to view images in the operating room during surgery to localize normal brain structures and tumor.

Several types of image-guided or **neuronavigation** systems are available to assist the neurosurgeon in localizing and removing the tumor during surgery. Some systems use magnetic resonance images taken before surgery together with special "markers" that are placed on the patient's head. The magnetic resonance images appear on a computer display in the operating room with the markers still in place corresponding to the exact location on the screen. The neurosurgeon can then use a special pointer to touch areas of the tumor that are seen on the patient's magnetic resonance imaging (MRI) scan. This allows the neurosurgeon to orient the instruments precisely during surgery, an advantage when the tumor is deep within the brain. Thus, a combination of direct visualization and corresponding MRI imaging may allow the neurosurgeon to remove more of the tumor safely.

Intraoperative MRI

An "MRI guidance" system available in operating rooms designed to function with an MRI scanner.

Another type of "MRI guidance" is **intraoperative MRI** (Color Plate 5), which is now available at many centers. These operating rooms are designed to function with an MRI scanner that can be used during the operation. As the neurosurgeon removes the tumor, the brain "sinks" away from the opening. This makes the residual tumor deeper and more difficult to visualize directly; therefore, an MRI scan taken during the procedure may allow the neurosurgeon to compensate for the "brain shift" that has occurred and see any remnants of tumor that remain. The neurosurgeon often checks a final MRI scan at the end of the operation, just to make sure that all of the tumor has been removed.

Remember, however, that many tumors can be safely removed or biopsied without the use of intraoperative MRI. Because intraoperative imaging takes more time, some neurosurgeons do not recommend it for peripheral or "surface" tumors. Some centers with intraoperative MRI have a waiting list. Discuss with your neurosurgeon whether referral for intraoperative MRI would be beneficial to you.

30. One of the people in my support group says that she had an "awake craniotomy" to remove her tumor. What is this procedure, and why did her neurosurgeon do this?

Some patients have a tumor near a critical area of the brain, such as the center that controls speech. Studies such as a functional MRI (see Question 24) can demonstrate the location of the speech center before the operation. During surgery, however, many tumors appear to blend into the surrounding normal brain, and thus, it is still possible to damage the speech center when attempting to remove the tumor completely.

In some hospitals and research centers, the patient is allowed to awaken after the neurosurgeon has opened the skull and dura, exposing the brain. The surface of the brain is covered with markers that identify which

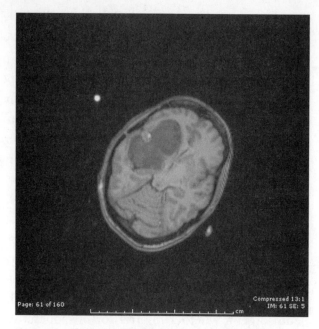

Figure 12   Intraoperative MRI image taken before surgery.

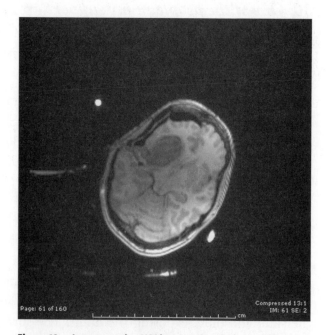

Figure 13   Intraoperative MRI image taken during surgery, showing a portion of the tumor removed.

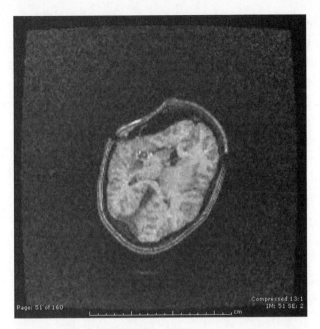

Figure 14   Intraoperative MRI image taken after the tumor has been completely resected. Photograph courtesy of Dr. Mike Desaloms, Dallas, Texas.

areas of the brain are involved in the production of speech. The patient may be given a series of words to read during surgery, but if stimulation of an area of the brain shows that the patient can no longer respond, the neurosurgeon knows that removing tumor from this area will most likely damage the speech center.

An awake craniotomy requires more time and preparation for the neurosurgeon and the operating team. Patients who may benefit from an awake craniotomy usually have tumors that can be completely resected or will respond to other therapy for any parts of the tumor that must be left behind.

How a Craniotomy Is Performed

A craniotomy ("cranio-" meaning skull and "-tomy" meaning incision) is the process of surgically "cutting" an opening into the skull. A craniotomy may be done

Neurosurgery

for a number of reasons, including repair of a blood vessel, removal of a blood clot, or removal (resection) of a tumor. Performing a craniotomy on a brain tumor patient is not necessarily synonymous with performing a resection. An open biopsy, for example, allows the neurosurgeon to visualize directly the surface of the brain before removing a piece of the tumor. A partial resection involves removing a larger portion of the tumor, and a gross total resection removes the entire visible tumor. All of these procedures begin by first removing enough of the skull to visualize the underlying brain and tumor.

This account describes what you would see during a craniotomy for gross total resection of a glioblastoma:

Before entering the operating room, the anesthesiologist sees the patient and inserts an intravenous catheter. A sedative is administered and the patient is taken to the operating room. The anesthesiologist and operating room nurses prepare the patient for surgery, placing the patient on the operating table and attaching monitors for temperature, heart rate, blood pressure, and oxygen saturation. The anesthesiologist inserts a hollow tube through the patient's mouth into the trachea that will deliver oxygen throughout the procedure while the patient is asleep.

The neurosurgeon and his assistants position the patient's head in a holder similar to a vise. The scalp overlying the site of the tumor is shaved, and the entire area is scrubbed with surgical soap. The rest of the head and body is covered with sterile surgical drapes.

The neurosurgeon cuts through the scalp with a scalpel, carefully cauterizing small bleeding vessels. The scalp and muscle flap created by the incision are peeled back to expose the skull. The edges of the flap are clamped and covered with a moist sterile cloth. A surgical drill is then placed against the surface of the skull, and four small holes are drilled, forming a square. A surgical saw is placed in one of the holes, and the four holes are connected, thus allowing a portion of the skull to be temporarily removed. This piece of skull is placed in a sterile salt solution until the end of the operation.

The tough, outermost membrane of the brain, the dura, is cut with scissors to fold back to the edges of the bone, exposing the surface of the brain. The tumor may be visible from the surface of the brain. A deeper tumor may be localized by ultrasound, intraoperative MRI, or another surgical navigation system. The neurosurgeon carefully cuts through the brain overlying the tumor until abnormal tissue is found. This tissue may appear different in color and texture from the surrounding normal brain. The neurosurgeon removes a small piece of the abnormal tissue for the pathologist to examine.

The pathologist prepares the tissue by freezing it in a small block and then slicing it into sections so that the tissue can be put onto microscope slides. These tiny pieces of tissue are then stained to reveal the structure of cells. Often, the pathologist can determine immediately whether tumor is present in the sample, whether the tumor is benign or malignant, and whether the tumor is primary or metastatic.

If the pathologist is able to make a diagnosis from the frozen section, the neurosurgeon is informed of the result. The neurosurgeon may remove additional pieces of the tumor for further analysis and permanent sections. If the neurosurgeon decides that it is too dangerous to remove additional tumor, the procedure is terminated; however, if the additional tumor can be safely removed or if the removal of large portions of the tumor will reduce pressure on the brain, the neurosurgeon may continue to remove as much of the tumor as possible. In some cases, the neurosurgeon may decide to insert chemotherapy wafers (Gliadel) in the tumor cavity. Gliadel contains a chemotherapy drug that penetrates into the surrounding brain tissue, to prevent regrowth of tumor cells that may still be present in the deeper areas adjacent to the tumor. The use of Gliadel depends on many factors, including the type of tumor, its size and its location.

The neurosurgeon and his assistant carefully inspect the brain for evidence of bleeding vessels, cauterizing them and bathing the exposed areas of the brain with sterile fluid. When the neurosurgeon is satisfied that all tumor tissue has been removed and that all bleeding has been controlled, the tumor cavity is filled with a sterile salt solution, and the dura is replaced over the brain. The dura is stitched with suture and checked for any tiny leaks along the suture line. The piece of skull removed at the beginning of the operation is then replaced, using small metal plates and screws, or other devices, to keep the skull piece in position. The muscle and scalp layers are then sutured together, and the free edges of the wound are finally sutured or stapled closed. A sterile dressing is then applied to the scalp.

The drapes are removed and the anesthesiologist prepares the patient for awakening. The breathing tube is removed, and the patient is taken to the recovery room.

M.L.'s comment:

Now that it's been several years since my surgery, reading this section does not bother me nearly as much as it previously did. When I think about the fact that this was done to me, it is still a bit unsettling, especially when I read that part about "a piece of my skull is placed in a sterile salt solution." I also had no idea that the cavity in my brain where the tumor used to be was filled up with "sterile salt solution." The part that was most sickening to me was the description of how everything is "stitched and stapled" back together. Somehow seeing neurosurgical procedures on television documentaries isn't quite the same as imagining that it's happened to your own head!

31. My neurosurgeon said that if I have a certain type of tumor, he could place Gliadel wafers in the brain after he removes the tumor, but he said that he won't know until surgery what type of tumor I have and that I have to decide before surgery whether I want him to do this. If I have Gliadel wafers placed during my surgery, can I still have chemotherapy?

Gliadel is a dissolvable wafer impregnated with a chemotherapy drug called carmustine (also known as BCNU). The wafer is designed to release chemotherapy slowly into the surrounding brain to treat microscopic tumor cells left behind after surgery. Gliadel was developed for malignant glial tumors, particularly glioblastoma, but has also been used for other primary brain tumors. If your surgeon is anticipating, based on your scans, that you have a malignant glioma, he may consider implanting Gliadel after he has resected the entire visible tumor. Gliadel wafers are placed up against the walls of the cavity where the tumor was removed, before closing the membranes, skull, and scalp (**Figures 15** and **16**).

> *Gliadel is a dissolvable wafer impregnated with a chemotherapy drug called carmustine (also known as BCNU). The wafer is designed to release chemotherapy slowly into the surrounding brain to treat microscopic tumor cells left behind after surgery.*

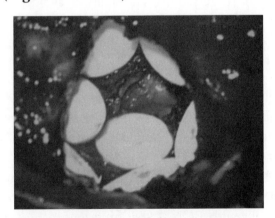

Figure 15 Gliadel wafers placed into the resection cavity following removal of the tumor. Photograph courtesy of Dr. Richard Weiner, Dallas, Texas.

87

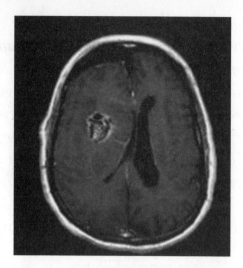

Figure 16   MRI image of Gliadel wafers in the resection cavity. Photograph courtesy of Dr. Richard Weiner, Dallas, Texas.

There are some possible side effects of Gliadel implantation. Although very little of the chemotherapy drug enters the bloodstream, it is still possible that chemotherapy leaking into the spinal fluid could affect how the wound heals if the neurosurgeon could not achieve a tight closure of the dura. It is also possible that Gliadel could increase the risk of seizures within a few days of surgery. This can usually be avoided by taking anticonvulsant medication. Finally, a few patients have more swelling of the surrounding brain at the site of the tumor resection when Gliadel has been used.

Gliadel releases chemotherapy into the brain for several days after surgery, but its effects are not permanent. Some patients have continued treatment with intravenous BCNU (the chemotherapy drug that is in the Gliadel wafer) after surgery. Although there is theoretically an advantage in continuing to treat any residual tumor cells with BCNU, the intravenous drug—unlike the chemotherapy wafer—affects blood counts and may cause other systemic toxicity. Clinical trials have studied the use of Gliadel followed by other drugs, including temozolomide (Temodar) and CPT-11 (Camptosar). There did not appear to be an increase in the expected side effects with these combinations.

Because Gliadel contains chemotherapy, some clinical trials for brain tumor treatment do not allow patients to participate if they have been previously treated with Gliadel. The patients in a clinical trial must all be similar. The trial results could be difficult to interpret if some patients had received Gliadel and others had not. If it is important to you to enter a clinical trial immediately after surgery, you should discuss this with your neurosurgeon before receiving Gliadel.

The randomized trials of patients with glioblastoma who received Gliadel have indicated, however, that long-term survival is improved, and long-term survival may be equal or better than the survival of patients who have had intravenous BCNU. Gliadel is often covered by insurance, but there is also a reimbursement program for patients who do not have insurance. You can find out more about Gliadel, as well as additional information about the brain and brain tumors, at their website at: www.gliadel.com.

32. At the time of my surgery, my neurosurgeon said that my entire tumor had been removed, but then he said that I would need more treatment to keep it from coming back. Why do I still need therapy if the malignant cells were removed?

Many common tumors, including astrocytomas, oligodendrogliomas, and lymphomas, may appear to be discrete, well-defined masses on an MRI. Occasionally, the neurosurgeon will observe a difference in the appearance of the tumor mass and the surrounding brain, but as a rule, these tumors tend to "blend in" and infiltrate the surrounding normal brain; therefore, the appearance on an MRI that the tumor is completely resectable may be misleading. The neurosurgeon may remove all clearly abnormal tissue, but he does not attempt to remove all of the microscopic tumor cells that have spread through the surrounding normal brain. Neurosurgeons who refer to a "gross total resection" are simply referring to their ability to remove all tissue that appeared to be part of the tumor.

Microscopic cells that have spread away from the main tumor mass, however, will continue to grow and must be treated. If the pathologist determines that the tumor is a type that will recur, follow-up treatment after surgery, such as radiation therapy or chemotherapy, is recommended.

33. On my most recent MRI, my neurosurgeon told me that my tumor is growing back. I asked him whether I should have surgery again, but he told me that he would have to discuss with my other doctors what treatment I could have after surgery. Why does treatment after surgery have an impact on whether I should have a second craniotomy?

As important as surgery is, it may only achieve partial control of a recurrent tumor. Just as radiation or chemotherapy may be important after the initial surgery, further therapy is usually recommended after a follow-up craniotomy. For many patients, conventional radiation therapy (see Question 35) cannot be repeated. Thus, if the tumor grows back after completing radiation therapy, another type of treatment should be used after a second surgery to control any microscopic tumor left behind; therefore, the benefit of a second surgery is likely to be temporary if another treatment cannot be found that would control the residual tumor. Also, your neurosurgeon may consider using Gliadel, even if it was not used for the initial surgery, since clinical trials have suggested that Gliadel delays recurrence following a second surgical resection.

34. My neurosurgeon suggested that I have physical therapy and occupational therapy to help me recover from my weakness after surgery. What is the difference between occupational therapy and physical therapy? Do I need both?

Achieving optimal neurological recovery after surgery may mean extensive rehabilitation. Rehabilitation programs are available in the inpatient and outpatient settings. Patients may receive rehabilitation while undergoing other treatments such as chemotherapy or radiation therapy.

Rehabilitation programs offer access to a variety of treatment professionals and specialized equipment to help patients receive a structured program for recovery. An initial evaluation by a neurologist specializing in rehabilitation or a **physiatrist**, a physician who specializes in physical medicine, is necessary to identify what should be included in the rehabilitation program. The rehabilitation program is customized to the patient's neurological deficits. Typically, brain tumor patients have a thorough evaluation to identify physical deficits as well as cognitive deficits; therefore, most patients benefit from a multidisciplinary program.

Physical therapy treats weakness, loss of coordination, and limited endurance. During physical therapy,

Physiatrist

Physician who specializes in physical medicine and rehabilitation and in prescribing the components of a rehabilitation program.

Physical therapy treats weakness, loss of coordination, and limited endurance.

Physical therapy

Therapy aimed at recovery from weakness, loss of coordination, or limited endurance.

Occupational therapy

Assists patients in normalizing activities of daily living, such as bathing, brushing teeth, cutting meat, and dressing.

Speech therapist

Professionals who evaluate speech production, speech comprehension, and swallowing function.

Recreational therapist

Assists patients to engage in leisure activities such as cooking, arts and crafts, and music therapy that can provide a cognitive component to the "work" of physical rehabilitation.

Rehabilitation counselor

Assesses the goals of the patient and his or her return to work and family life.

Neuropsychologist

Professionals who specialize in the effect of brain injury on behavior and cognition. They help identify ways to improve relearning and to compensate for neurological functions that are impaired.

patients learn to walk unassisted, to use a cane or walker, or to transfer safely from the bed to a chair or wheelchair. Patients may be fitted with a brace or other supportive device to compensate for weak or stiff limbs. Activities may begin while the patient is still confined to bed recovering from surgery because even passive movement of the limbs helps prevent complications such as blood clots and bedsores. **Occupational therapy** assists the patient in performing activities of daily living, such as bathing, brushing teeth, cutting food, and dressing. Occupational therapists may use recreational activities such as puzzles to help patients improve their hand–eye coordination and cognitive function.

Other treatment professionals that may be needed in a rehabilitation program include **speech therapists**, **recreational therapists**, **rehabilitation counselors**, and **neuropsychologists**. Speech therapists evaluate speech production and comprehension. In addition, speech therapists work with patients who have difficulty swallowing. Recreational therapists engage patients in leisure activities, such as cooking, arts and crafts, and music therapy. These activities provide "play" to balance the "work" of physical rehabilitation. Rehabilitation counselors assess the goals of the patient in relationship to the return to work and family life. Neuropsychologists specialize in the effect of brain injury on behavior and cognition. They help identify ways to relearn certain skills as well as advise patients on how to compensate for neurological functions that are impaired.

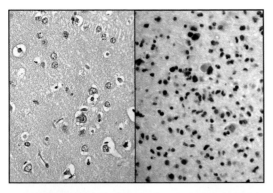

1. The image on the left is normal brain and the image on the right is a low grade glioma. Note that the low grade glioma has many more cells, but they are fairly uniform. Blood vessels in both specimens are normal.

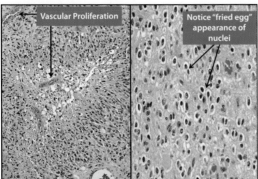

Vascular Proliferation

Notice "fried egg" appearance of nuclei

2. The image on the left is a glioblastoma, one of the most common primary brain tumors. It is a high grade, rapidly growing tumor, characterized by large numbers of cells that vary in size and shape; proliferation of blood vessels; and areas of "necrosis" (or dying cells). The adjacent image is a low grade oligodendroglioma, characterized by round cell nuclei with a clear "halo."

Plates 1 and 2: *Reproduced from Dr. K. Hatantaa, M.D., Neuropathologist, University of Texas Southwestern Medical School, Dallas, TX.*

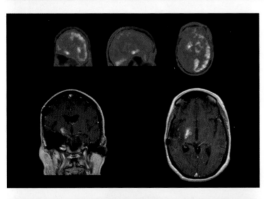

3. PET/MRI showing both low intensity at the site of radiotherapy and high intensity at the site of recurrences. The blue and purple areas on the left half of the image show less glucose uptake than normal because this area was previously radiated. The small enhanced (white) area on MRI corresponds to an area of increased glucose uptake (yellow) on the PET. This is consistent with a recurrence of tumor.

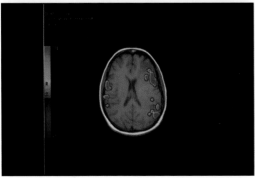

4. Functional MRI. Functional MRI is an image created by increased blood flow, as the highlighted portion of the brain is "functioning." Areas involved in speech, motor function, and other activities can be mapped as the patient is asked to perform certain tasks. The spots of color in the image show regions of high uptake.

5. Intraoperative MRI using BrainSUITE® iMRI imaging technology.

Image Courtesy of Brain–LAB AG.

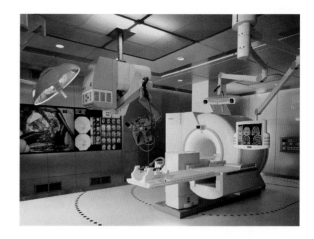

6. Computer-generated image of an area in the brain to be treated with radiotherapy (RT). Such images are used in planning RT treatment. The colors represent the target area (red) and relative doses of radiation away from the target (yellow, pink, green, and blue lines).

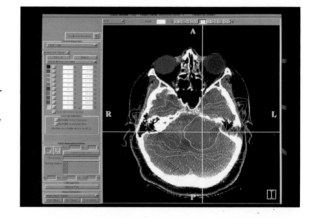

7. Tumors get their blood supply by releasing vascular endothelial growth factors (VEGFs). VEGFs attach to receptors in existing blood vessels, which stimulates new blood vessel growth. Anti-VEGF agents, such as Avastin, bind with the VEGFs and block them from connecting to the receptors. This prevents new blood vessel growth, eventually starving the tumor.

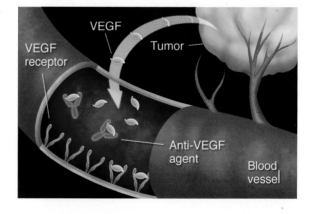

PART FIVE

Radiation Therapy

What is radiation therapy? Is radiation therapy given for every type of brain tumor?

What are the side effects of radiation therapy?

How does the radiation oncologist decide how much of the brain to radiate if nothing is visible on the MRI?

More . . .

35. What is radiation therapy? Is radiation therapy given for every type of brain tumor?

To kill a cancer cell, it is necessary to interfere with its ability to grow and divide and form more cancer cells. A form of energy called **ionizing radiation** creates a high enough energy to knock the electrons in the molecules of living cells out of their normal orbits. This creates enough energy to disrupt other nearby electrons, which in turn affects the deoxyribonucleic acid (DNA) of the cell. Radiation can cause breaks in the strands of DNA, causing cell injury and eventually cell death. Both X-rays and gamma rays are forms of ionizing radiation.

Radiation therapy uses X-rays, a man-made form of ionizing radiation, to penetrate through tissue into a tumor. A **linear accelerator** is one machine that produces such radiation. The linear accelerator delivers **external beam radiation** (also known as conventional radiation) (**Figure 17**).

Ionizing radiation

A form of energy that knocks electrons out of their normal orbits.

Linear accelerator

A machine used in radiation therapy that is able to create man-made ionizing radiation in the form of X-rays to penetrate through tissue into a tumor.

External beam radiation

The type of radiation therapy delivered by a linear accelerator.

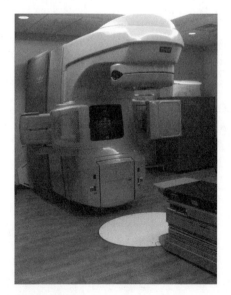

Figure 17   Linear accelerator.
Source: Timothy Nichols, M.D., Northpoint Cancer Center.

Both normal cells and cancer cells can repair radiation cellular damage to a variable degree. By dividing the dose of radiation into small daily doses called **fractions**, normal cells are relatively spared because they are better able to repair DNA damage. Most cancer cells, however, lack the ability to repair DNA damage completely, and over the course of several days of treatment, the cancer cells will die. The amount of radiation energy absorbed by the body is measured in **Gray**. The amount of radiation used in cancer therapy is typically divided in hundredths of a Gray, called **centiGray**, abbreviated cGy. An older term sometimes used in radiation measurement is the rad, which is equal to 1 cGy.

Not all brain tumors are treated with radiation therapy, and different types of brain tumors require different radiation **target volumes** (the volume of brain tissue to be treated). For example, multiple small tumors throughout the brain, which commonly occur in metastatic lung cancer, are usually treated with **whole-brain radiation therapy**. This therapy is also used for primary brain tumors that have multiple tumors present at the same time, including primary central nervous system (CNS) lymphoma. Most primary brain tumors, which occur as a single abnormality on an MRI scan (magnetic resonance imaging), are treated with radiation therapy directed at the tumor and a margin of 2 or 3 centimeters around it. This treatment approach is called local or partial brain radiation therapy. Sometimes the central portion of the tumor is treated with a high dose of fractionated radiation called a **boost**.

Tumors vary in their **radiosensitivity**, which means that some are easy to control with the standard doses of radiation therapy and some shrink little or not at all.

Radiation Therapy

Fraction
Single treatment of radiation.

Gray (Gy)
Modern unit of radiation dosage.

CentiGray (cGy)
Unit of radiation, equal to one rad.

Target volume
The three-dimensional portion of an organ or organs, identified from the patient's scans or X-rays, to receive radiation therapy treatments.

Whole-brain radiation therapy
Radiation therapy delivered to the entire intracranial contents.

Boost
High dose of fractionated radiation.

Radiosensitivity
A tumor's susceptibility to growth inhibition or cell killing by radiation therapy.

Stereotactic radiation

Type of radiation therapy that focuses energy to a small area of a tumor, usually less than 3 to 4 centimeters in diameter. It may be fractionated over several treatments.

Gamma Knife radiation therapy uses a special radiation unit that is designed to deliver radiation from multiple cobalt sources.

Stereotactic radiosurgery (SRS)

A radiation therapy technique using a large number of narrow, precisely aimed, highly focused beams of ionizing radiation. Beams aimed from many directions meet at a specific point. Usually only one treatment at a high dose is planned.

Cobalt

A radioactive isotope used in the treatment of cancer.

After surgical resection, some types of tumors will begin to grow back if any microscopic tumor is left behind. For these tumors, radiation may be used to prevent this microscopic disease from recurring in the area around the resected tumor. Other tumors cannot be removed completely because of their location, and radiation becomes the primary mode of treatment.

Additional types of radiation therapy include **stereotactic radiation** and **stereotactic radiosurgery** (SRS). These approaches focus radiation energy to a small area of tumor (usually less than 3 to 4 centimeters in diameter). These therapies do not involve surgery, but they do have "surgical precision."

One type of stereotactic radiosurgery is called Gamma Knife. Gamma Knife radiation therapy uses a special radiation unit that is designed to deliver radiation from multiple **cobalt** sources. Gamma Knife is most commonly used to treat small metastatic tumors. It may also be used to treat other small benign tumors such as acoustic neuromas, meningiomas, and pituitary tumors. Stereotactic radiosurgery is delivered with one single large dose, 15 to 30 Gy (10 times the usual daily dose for fractionated radiation therapy). Both Gamma Knife and other types of stereotactic radiosurgery use some type of frame or fixation to keep the patient exactly in position during treatment.

Other types of **stereotactic radiotherapy** also use highly localized radiation, and doses are divided into fractions over a few days. In this case, the frame or fixation used still keeps the patient in an exact location, but can be removed between treatments.

Brachytherapy delivers radiation therapy from the inside of the tumor to the surrounding area. The radiation can be delivered in several different ways. Sometimes radioactive pellets or seeds are implanted. Sometimes removable sources of radiation are used. Sometimes radioactive liquid is inserted into the tumor cavity or into a balloon catheter that is surgically inserted into the tumor. Radioactive isotopes have also been linked to monoclonal antibodies to the tumor cells in an effort to direct radiation therapy more specifically to spare normal cells.

What to Expect during Radiation Therapy

Patients who will receive radiation therapy as part of their treatment for a primary or metastatic brain tumor meet with a radiation oncologist, a doctor who specializes in treating tumors with radiation therapy. Although a radiation oncologist may visit with you after surgery while you are still in the hospital, most radiation therapy is conducted on an outpatient basis.

After discussing the potential benefits and risks of radiation therapy, the radiation oncologist discusses the detailed treatment plan, and the patient signs an **informed consent**. This explains potential risks and complications of the treatment.

The patient's MRI or computed tomography (CT) scans are reviewed by the radiation oncologist to determine the target volume (the area that will be irradiated). Sometimes additional microscopic tumor cells grow at the edge of the tumor visualized on brain scans. The radiation oncologist takes this into account by including a margin of 1 to 3 centimeters around the tumor in the target volume. The radiation oncologist also notes sensitive areas that should not receive full doses of radiation, such as the eyes or the brain stem.

The radiation oncologist and the **radiation physicist** determine the doses of radiation that the patient will

Radiation Therapy

Stereotactic radiotherapy

Type of radiation therapy that focuses the dose to a small area of a tumor, usually less than 3 to 4 centimeters in diameter, fractionated over a few days.

Brachytherapy

Internal radiation therapy that involves placing radioactive material near or in the tumor.

Informed consent

Process of explaining to the patient all risks and complications of a procedure or treatment before it is done. Informed consents are signed by the patient, a parent of a minor child, or a legal representative.

Radiation physicist

A scientist trained to determine the dose and accuracy of radiation therapy equipment.

receive. They calculate the total amount of radiation to the tumor as well as the amount that will be distributed over the remaining portions of the brain. With conventional radiation therapy, areas adjacent to the tumor receive a percentage of the total dose (Color Plate 6). With other forms of radiation therapy, such as radiosurgery, the areas adjacent to the tumor receive no radiation. To make sure that the patient receives the dose in exactly the same configuration day after day, the radiation technicians create a custom "mask" that holds the patient firmly in place. This is often a mold or a net-like device that allows the patient to breathe normally but still holds the head in place during treatment.

Simulation

A practice treatment that allows the radiation team to determine exactly where the radiation treatment will be directed.

With the patient in position, X-rays may be taken to provide a **simulation** of the exact target volume. When the radiation oncologist is satisfied with the treatment planning, the actual treatment begins. The treatment session, once planning is completed, is typically brief, often lasting about 15 minutes.

During treatment, the linear accelerator, a source of radiation therapy, rotates around the patient very precisely. Different angles may be used, from the sides of the head or front to back, to focus intersecting beams of radiation at the tumor. The treatment may be modified during radiation therapy if a smaller section of the tumor will receive a "boost." This may require more CT or MRI planning and a second planning session.

Typically, the radiation oncologist sees the patient at least weekly during treatment. The radiation oncologist may recommend treatment with steroids if the patient develops symptoms of swelling around the tumor during radiation therapy such as a headache or a pressure sensation. Any other side effects of treatment are also discussed with the radiation oncologist.

After completing radiation therapy, the radiation oncologist reviews the posttreatment MRI with the patient. Because of changes in the tumor and surrounding tissue that may occur during radiation therapy, the MRI is usually evaluated several weeks after radiation therapy ends; however, the tumor may continue to shrink for several months after the completion of radiation therapy, and thus, additional scans are often recommended to assess the success of treatment.

M.L.'s comment:

After my craniotomy, my neurosurgeon and radiation oncologist recommended further treatment with radiation therapy. Additional treatments with chemotherapy were also recommended, but I didn't start them until after my radiation treatments (although now many patients do chemotherapy and radiation therapy simultaneously). Even though my neurosurgeon had indicated that he had been able to remove the visible tumor, it was likely that some cancer cells remained. Those cells needed to be treated with radiation therapy.

The treatments didn't hurt at all. I think the most uncomfortable part of my regular radiation treatments was having the "mask" made for my head and face. I had to lie still (and I mean still) for what seemed like forever while a plastic mesh-like form was molded to my head and face. This was done so that the radiation oncologist could mark in ink the locations where the radiation beams would be targeted every single time that I had a treatment. Before having the technology to make these masks, it's my understanding that the radiation oncologist would make these marks on your skin, and these marks don't just come off with soap and water. Needless to say, the mask is certainly the preferred method, but having to lay still for so long hurt the back of my head a lot more than the regular radiation treatments ever did.

When I refer to "regular" radiation treatments, I'm talking about the daily "conventional" treatments that I received every day for 6 weeks. I did, however, have additional radiation therapy called stereotactic radiosurgery, but it wasn't the Gamma Knife procedure. The stereotactic radio-surgery that I received had recently been developed and was called the m3. It was developed by BrainLAB. The m3 allows precisely focused, high-dose X-ray beams to be delivered to a very small area of the brain.

With m3, special planning with the computer allows a large dose of radiation to be delivered to the tumor site with minimal radiation going to the normal or "good" brain tissue that surrounds the tumor site. In my situation, the radiosurgery was delivered as a local "boost" after my 6 weeks of regular or conventional radiation.

This procedure isn't painful; however, you should be pre-pared for the fact that you have to wear what the doctors call a halo. It's a metal frame that is placed on your head and attached with screws in four places: two in the back of your head and two in the front. The halo ensures that your head doesn't move during the treatment. The doctors put a topical anesthetic on so that the screws don't hurt too much as the halo is being attached. I also received pain medica-tion, which helped. After the frame was attached, I had a CT scan. The results of that were paired up with the results of the MRI that I had received 2 days before. By doing this, the medical team that was performing this procedure was able to pinpoint the exact size, shape, and location of the affected area as well as plot the dose of radiation that I would receive that day. The amount of radiation that I received the day of my radiosurgery was almost as much radiation as I would have received during an entire week of conventional treatment. The actual treatment only took about an hour, but the whole process took the entire day because the planning procedure took about 6 hours.

I will say that the most painful part was when the halo was removed. I think the pain medication had worn off, and when the screws were removed, I experienced a terrible wave of pain in my head. It was like having a terrible headache all of a sudden. It didn't last too long, but that was the only time that the "halo" actually felt more like a "crown of thorns!" If you undergo this procedure, you should make sure that you have been given enough pain medication so that when the halo is removed you don't have to experience the same kind of pain that I experienced.

My radiation oncologist said that the headache I experienced after the frame was removed is common. It's caused by a sudden drop in intracranial pressure. The frame produces an intense pressure on the skull, equivalent to 80 pounds per square inch. This pressure on the skull deforms the skull during the hours that the frame is in place. The amount of spinal fluid actually decreases in volume in response to the pressure on the skull. When the frame is taken off, the skull springs back, causing a sudden drop in spinal fluid pressure and an intense headache. Aside from that one painful moment, I do NOT regret having this procedure because it was the end result that was most important.

36. What are the side effects of radiation therapy?

Several factors influence the risk of developing side effects from radiation therapy. They include the total volume of the brain irradiated, the location of the radiation fields, the total dose received, and the age of the patient. These factors vary from patient to patient.

Radiation side effects may also vary over the course of time. Cells that grow relatively quickly, including those of the skin and hair follicles, are affected relatively quickly, often during the course of radiation. Hair loss in the area of the scalp overlying the tumor is typical.

Radiation side effects may also vary over the course of time.

Patients who receive whole-brain radiation therapy may have almost total loss of hair, but the use of modern radiation equipment that "shapes" the target volume tends to spare the scalp so that hair loss is rarely permanent.

Other types of cells, including the normal glial cells of the brain and the blood vessels, are affected months to years after radiation. Occasionally, patients complain of fatigue, weakness, or feeling mentally "foggy" during and for several weeks after radiation therapy. These side effects are quite variable in their severity and duration. Despite these side effects, many patients are able to continue their normal activities.

Some long-term side effects that often concern patients bear special mention. Patients are often concerned about short-term memory loss or cognitive changes after radiation therapy. Again, the volume of brain irradiated, the areas of the brain irradiated, the total dose received, and the age of the patient are factors that impact the cognitive changes that are observed at least 1 year after treatment. The use of chemotherapy during radiation may also be associated with cognitive changes. Although the best studies of the effects of whole-brain radiation therapy on cognition, as measured by IQ testing, have been done in children, there is ample evidence to suggest that adults can suffer cognitive loss, particularly in short-term memory, after whole-brain radiation therapy. Although partial-brain irradiation has also shown some effect on cognition, the effects tend to be less pronounced and may take longer to become apparent.

A second long-term side effect that may affect patients who have received relatively high-dose radiation therapy is **radiation necrosis**. Radiation necrosis is an area of injured normal glial cells and blood vessels. It can occur anywhere from several months to 2 to 3 years after radiation therapy. The appearance of radiation necrosis on an MRI may be indistinguishable from tumor recurrence. There is typically an area of enhancement, surrounded by edema, and the area may even appear to enlarge over subsequent scans. Patients experiencing radiation necrosis may develop neurological symptoms such as weakness, loss of coordination, or visual disturbances that may mimic tumor recurrence. Surgery may be required to remove the area of necrosis. Radiation necrosis is more common after high doses of focused radiation therapy, such as radiosurgery or brachytherapy.

Radiation necrosis

An area of injured normal glial cells and blood vessels that may occur several months after radiation therapy.

Because radiation therapy affects the blood vessels within the radiation field, there is potential for cerebral vascular injury. In the majority of patients, only very small blood vessels are affected, and injury of these vessels typically does not cause symptoms; however, some blood vessels may be severely narrowed, and stroke-like symptoms may occur. Patients who have other risk factors for stroke such as high blood pressure, high cholesterol, and diabetes may wish to discuss these conditions with their radiation oncologist.

Secondary malignancy

Cancer that develops as a result of previous cancer therapy.

Another complication of radiation therapy, although rare, may occur several years after treatment. A **secondary malignancy** is a cancer that develops as a result of previous cancer therapy. Secondary malignancies may occur in patients who have received curative radiation therapy for childhood or early adulthood brain tumors or may occur after whole-brain radiation therapy for acute leukemia. The original tumor has not recurred, but a new type of tumor (often a malignant glioma) appears within the radiation field. The risk of secondary malignant tumors 15 years after radiation therapy is estimated at less than 5%; however, a secondary malignant tumor may be more difficult to treat, as the patient has previously had radiation therapy to the same area. In addition to secondary malignancies, benign tumors, including meningiomas and nerve sheath tumors, may also develop after radiation therapy.

M.L.'s comment:

The side effects that I experienced during radiation were primarily fatigue and hair loss. Some days the fatigue was greater than others, but I soon realized that I needed to just give in to the fact that I was tired and needed to take a nap; however, a nap or a good night's sleep may not always relieve your fatigue. It's very common for cancer patients to experience fatigue, and it can affect you in many ways other than just feeling tired or weary. In addition to not having as much energy during the day, I experienced periods of depression. I would begin to cry whenever I would talk to a loved one, especially my mother or sister. Because they both live far away, I felt sort of alone. I really wasn't alone, though. In fact, I had an overwhelming amount of support and comfort throughout the worst part of my treatments. Despite such support, I found that I couldn't help crying at times. In my case, this feeling of depression didn't go on too long.

If you find that you're having a difficult time with fatigue, there are things that you can do to minimize the feelings of fatigue and frustration. Try to remember to rest when you feel like you need it; don't fight the fatigue. Also, try to eat right. Eat foods that will give you energy. Your doctors should be able to give you some helpful ideas of what you should and shouldn't eat. Try to get some sort of exercise every day, even if it's just a short walk around the block. I found that just getting outside and getting a bit of fresh air every day helped to relieve some of the fatigue that I was feeling. Finally, don't forget to have some sort of a social life. Just because you have a brain tumor doesn't mean that you have to stop having fun. A reduction in your social life will help to conserve some of your energy, but you shouldn't feel like you have to cut out all of the things that you enjoy doing. It's all about being able to prioritize and balance what you must do in order to keep from being too tired.

37. My tumor was completely resected, but I understand that there could still be microscopic tumor left behind. How does the radiation oncologist decide how much of the brain to radiate if nothing is visible on the MRI?

Several years ago, studies of patients with malignant gliomas who received whole-brain radiation therapy showed that tumor recurrence frequently occurred within 2 to 5 centimeters of the original site. Those studies also found that new tumors separate and distant from the original tumor occurred in only about 5% of patients; therefore, most radiation for malignant glioma (and many other solitary primary brain tumors) is now limited to the area of the tumor and a margin around the tumor.

The MRI scans performed before surgery help to determine how much area around the tumor cavity should be included in the radiation field. For tumors that infiltrate into the surrounding brain, a margin of at least 2 centimeters around the tumor is often recommended. Well-circumscribed tumors may require a smaller margin, and tumors with extensive surrounding edema may require a larger margin. Clinical trials that include radiation therapy often specify how the radiation field will be designed and the margin that will be used.

There are exceptions, however! Primary CNS lymphoma, germinoma, and many metastatic brain tumors have a high risk of recurrence if treated with only a limited, or partial brain, treatment volume. These tumors tend to be microscopically more diffuse throughout the brain than they appear on an MRI. Because both the short- and long-term side effects of whole-brain radiation therapy are more severe, many research trials have tried to eliminate the need for whole-brain radiation therapy where feasible. For primary CNS lymphoma, several trials have demonstrated that systemic intravenous chemotherapy, or intra-arterial chemotherapy, have results equivalent or superior to treatment plans that incorporate whole-brain radiation therapy (see Part Six). In the case of metastatic tumors, patients may elect to have follow-up scans at frequent intervals and treat any new tumors that appear with stereotactic radiosurgery or Gamma Knife (although this is not always possible or practical if the metastases are very large or numerous).

If you are concerned about receiving whole-brain radiation therapy, you may wish to investigate whether you are eligible for another type of therapy or a clinical trial that limits the use of whole-brain radiation.

38. What is the difference between stereotactic radiosurgery, CyberKnife, and Gamma Knife? How does my doctor determine which is appropriate for me?

Stereotactic radiosurgery (SRS), Gamma Knife, and CyberKnife are all forms of highly **conformal radiation therapy**; Gamma Knife and CyberKnife are specific *types* of stereotactic radiosurgery. Conformal means that the target volume is very well defined, or shaped, to the tumor or other lesion to be radiated. This requires that the patient is fixed firmly in position during the treatment so that the exact size and shape of the target volume is maintained for minutes or even hours. Gamma Knife and most other forms of linear accelerator-based SRS systems use a frame or rigid mask to immobilize the patient during this critical period. CyberKnife, in contrast, is a "frameless" SRS system. All of these radiosurgery procedures are performed by a team of neurosurgeons, radiation oncologists, and radiation physicists.

Stereotactic radiosurgery can be performed by a linear accelerator (linac) modified to produce a beam of photons to a small (less than 3 to 4 cm) tumor. The fixation of the patient's head in a stereotactic frame enables the radiation source to move around the target over a period of minutes, delivering a single high dose. Computer imaging can direct the beam to conform to the shape of the tumor. With some types of fixation systems, the dose can also be fractionated over several treatments; it is then called stereotactic radiotherapy.

Gamma Knife uses cobalt as a radiation source. The radiation sources are symmetrically arranged in a helmet-like pattern over the patient's head (**Figures 18a and b**). The

Stereotactic radiosurgery (SRS), Gamma Knife, and CyberKnife are all forms of highly conformal radiation therapy; Gamma Knife and CyberKnife are specific types of stereotactic radiosurgery.

Conformal radiation therapy

Three-dimensional radiation using images from a CT scan and an MRI to plan precise fields of radiation that may be contoured around structures such as the eyes or the brainstem.

Radiation Therapy

Gamma Knife Machine and Helmet

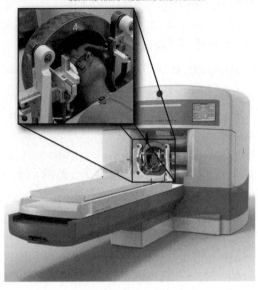

Figure 18a   Gamma Knife machine.

Source: Courtesy of Elekta, Inc.

radiation beams converge on the target with a high degree of accuracy, but the radiation sources do not move. Gamma Knife is not fractionated, but multiple lesions can be treated in the same setting, if necessary.

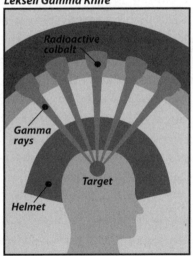

Figure 18b   How Gamma Knife targets a tumor.

Source: NRC File Photo.

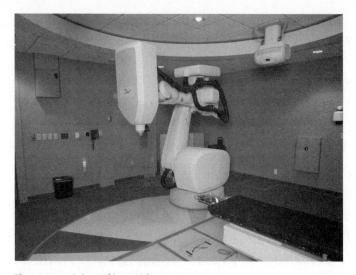

Figure 19   CyberKnife machine.
Source: Peter Lanasa, M.D., USMD CyberKnife Center.

The CyberKnife (**Figure 19**) uses a combination of robotics and image guidance to locate and track the position of the tumor without the use of a head frame. Because the patient is constantly imaged, the linear accelerator located within the highly flexible robotic arm can continue to treat the tumor even when the patient is moving. CyberKnife may also be preferred if a patient has had recent brain surgery because the pressure caused by the frame is avoided. It can be used to treat tumors in other difficult-to-reach locations, such as the spinal cord and lung.

Both linac-based SRS and Gamma Knife are best suited for small, spherical tumors, particularly metastases and acoustic neuromas. Gamma Knife is also used to treat vascular malformations and other nontumor conditions in the brain.

Most patients will have access to a center with Gamma Knife or SRS. Your doctor may prefer one type of treatment over the other for your specific type of tumor. More information regarding Gamma Knife

109

or SRS treatment will be available at your initial evaluation with your radiation oncologist.

39. I have an anaplastic astrocytoma that was treated 4 years ago with radiation therapy. Last week, for the first time, my MRI showed two new areas of tumor, each about an inch in diameter. My radiation oncologist and neurosurgeon said that I could have Gamma Knife to "zap" them; however, I have been reading a lot on the Internet, and it seems that my tumor is not usually treated with Gamma Knife. Why not?

In this case, you have hit on a controversial issue where experts do not always agree. A randomized study of radiosurgery in glioma that added a radiosurgery "boost" to half of the patients treated with conventional radiation therapy and chemotherapy actually showed no improvement in survival and increased toxicity in the patients receiving the boost; nevertheless, some radiation oncologists believe that there are some high-grade glioma patients who do benefit from a very precise, high dose of radiation to small areas of recurrent tumor. This does not substitute for external beam radiation therapy; it is typically done after radiation therapy.

Most high-grade gliomas, including your tumor type, anaplastic astrocytoma, are not "small." Tumors that appear distinct and well circumscribed on an MRI are often much larger than they appear to be because of the extension of microscopic cells around the "borders" of the tumor. For this reason, estimating the tumor to be "an inch in diameter" is likely to underestimate the true extent of the tumor. A large treatment perimeter planned for such tumors will "zap" more normal cells with a high dose, resulting in a risk of radiation necrosis. A small treatment perimeter, however, will not treat enough cells, and most tumors treated in this way will continue to grow at the margins.

On the other hand, some radiation oncologists and neurosurgeons who specialize in stereotactic radiosurgery are careful to point out that some patients seem to derive benefit and that radiosurgery is fast, usually well-tolerated, and avoids more toxic therapy such as systemic chemotherapy. In some cases, a combination of chemotherapy and stereotactic radiation therapy may be used. Although the toxicity is higher, this approach is intended to treat the visible tumor as well as the microscopic tumor outside the target volume.

As with most other issues in neuro-oncology, your case may be reviewed by another specialist before you have to make a final decision. If possible, try to consult a radiation oncologist who has extensive experience in Gamma Knife and who follows patients for several years after treatment. The website: www.virtualtrials.com lists physicians who will review your history and scans at no charge and try to assist you in finding your best treatment option.

40. I have seen two radiation oncologists. One says that he uses three-dimensional imaging to plan treatment. He says this targets the tumor more precisely, which makes the treatment safer. The other radiation oncologist says that only the total dose of radiation determines the extent of side effects. Who's right?

Both doctors are right. When a patient undergoes radiation therapy, the total dose of radiation delivered must not exceed safe parameters, and radiation delivery must avoid those sensitive brain structures that are not affected by the tumor. Conformal radiation therapy, a three-dimensional radiation treatment, uses images from a CT or an MRI scan to plan precise fields of radiation that can be contoured around sensitive structures such as the eyes or the brainstem. By using conformal radiation therapy, the total radiation dose delivered to the tumor may be the same as conventional external-beam radiation therapy, but the dose delivered to the surrounding normal brain may be less.

Many radiation facilities now have intensity-modulated radiation therapy (IMRT), which uses computer-controlled intensity modulation of the radiation beam during treatment. The radiation oncologist also uses "inverse treatment planning," specifying areas to avoid, as well as allowing multiple small fields to be treated simultaneously. Combinations of several intensity-modulated fields coming from different directions allow a very precise radiation dose to the target volume, as nearby normal structures receive much less. It is important, with such precision, to keep the patient precisely oriented during treatment, as movement will potentially expose normal tissue to more radiation than intended.

Using image-guided radiation therapy and intensity-modulated radiation therapy, radiation oncologists at some centers have the ability to administer a single dose of radiation high enough to destroy the cancer without affecting the spinal cord.

This problem is now being addressed by another new radiation technique, image-guided radiation therapy (IGRT). Using this technology (sometimes called four-dimensional radiation therapy), a tumor can be imaged just before the delivery of radiotherapy or even during a treatment, compensating for tumor movement. This is particularly important in tumors of the spine because the spinal cord is more susceptible to radiation damage than the brain. Using image-guided radiation therapy and intensity-modulated radiation therapy, radiation oncologists at some centers have the ability to administer a single dose of radiation high enough to destroy the cancer without affecting the spinal cord.

41. My doctor told me that I have a rare tumor, a chordoma, which is near the base of the skull. He suggested that I consider proton beam therapy. What is proton beam therapy, and why is it used?

In **proton beam therapy**, protons are accelerated with a particle accelerator onto the tumor. Because of their large mass, protons can be focused on the tumor shape and deliver their energy over a precise range and depth. All protons of a given energy have the same range, and the maximum dose delivered is over the last few millimeters of the particle's range. This maximum is called the Bragg peak, and the particles are accelerated to the desired depth of the tumor. The sharp cutoff edge of the dose is a distinct advantage for relatively superficial tumors such as salivary gland tumors, ocular tumors, and chordomas.

Proton beam therapy has achieved a significant improvement in the control of chordomas and chondrosarcomas near the base of the skull and upper cervical cord. These tumors are typically near critical structures such as the brainstem, spinal cord, and optic nerves. Because of the lower radiation dose to surrounding structures, protons have less severe side effects than conventional radiation therapy.

Proton beam therapy, also known as particle beam therapy, is available at only a few centers in the United States because of the need for expensive, heavy equipment such as cyclotrons and synchrocyclotrons. Today, there are proton beam centers operating or opening soon in several cities, including Loma Linda, California; Oklahoma City, Oklahoma; Houston, Texas; Boston, Massachusetts; Hampton, Virginia; Seattle, Washington; and St. Louis, Missouri.

Proton beam therapy

A cancer therapy that uses a beam of protons to irradiate a tumor while minimizing damage to surrounding healthy tissue.

Radiation Therapy

42. What is interstitial brachytherapy?

Interstitial brachytherapy

Radiation therapy that is administered from the inside of the tumor cavity, with a source of radiation therapy such as radioactive iodine or iridium.

Interstitial brachytherapy (interstitial = within space, brachy = short) refers to radiation therapy that is administered from the inside of the tumor cavity. Sources of radiation include iodine or iridium. In this treatment approach, radioactive seeds or pellets are implanted directly into the tumor cavity. The seeds or pellets deliver a low dose of radiation continuously to nearby surrounding tissue. Another type of brachytherapy uses a radioisotope, sometimes linked to a monoclonal antibody, injected directly into the tumor cavity or a balloon inserted into the cavity. Patients who are suitable candidates for brachytherapy have a well-circumscribed, resectable tumor less than 5 centimeters in diameter. All of these techniques deliver radiation therapy "from the inside out."

Although in some studies brachytherapy has been associated with an improvement in overall survival, some patients have needed another operation to remove radiation necrosis.

43. I had a biopsy of a tumor in my left hemisphere that measures 2 × 2 centimeters. The biopsy determined the tumor was a low-grade astrocytoma. I have seen a radiation oncologist who suggested immediate radiation therapy. When I got a second opinion from another radiation oncologist, he suggested that radiation therapy could be delayed for a few years. Why are the recommendations so different?

Treatment recommendations for brain tumors, particularly for low-grade gliomas, are guided by many factors. To help guide treatment decisions, many doctors refer to practice guidelines. The National Comprehensive Cancer Network (NCCN), a committee composed of neuro-oncologists, radiation oncologists, and neurosurgeons around the country, publishes such practice guidelines. The NCCN practice guidelines provide treatment recommendations that are based on current cancer research as well as the clinical experience of the committee members.

Many physicians use the NCCN guidelines as a reference, but many do not. Some academic centers and research institutions have developed their own guidelines for the treatment of specific brain tumors; however, all practice guidelines assume that doctors exercise good medical judgment in the patient's care, taking into consideration the patient's age and general health. Even the NCCN recommendations are not a "cookbook" approach for the treatment of any type of brain tumor. This is why different doctors may have different recommendations for treatment. Practice guidelines provide doctors with information that help to guide treatment, but the factors involved in your specific case also impact treatment decisions.

Low-grade gliomas can be quite variable in their behavior, making general recommendations difficult. Some gliomas are surgically resectable, but others spread into the surrounding brain and cannot be removed safely. If the tumor can be completely resected, some studies have shown that survival improves. Other studies have demonstrated that aggressive surgical resection does not improve survival.

Radiation therapy is often recommended for patients with low-grade gliomas that cannot be resected; however, because some patients have few, if any, symptoms, their doctors may recommend delaying radiation therapy until symptoms develop or until there is a change in the appearance of the tumor on an MRI scan. Again, clinical trials have shown conflicting results on which approach (immediate or delayed radiation) makes a difference in overall survival.

At least 50% of low-grade astrocytomas do become more malignant over a period of several years, progressing to anaplastic astrocytoma (Grade 3) or glioblastoma multiforme (Grade 4). This change can occur whether or not the patient has received radiation therapy; however, patients who have previously received a full course of radiation therapy may not be able to receive more radiation if the tumor recurs as a higher-grade tumor. Also, radiation can increase the risk of developing a second tumor, but this risk is considered very small (probably less than 5% within 15 years after radiation).

Although neither group of physicians you have seen recommended chemotherapy, some clinical trials have studied regimens such as PCV (Procarbazine, CCNU, and Vincristine) or Temodar in low-grade glioma patients with or without radiation therapy. It is not yet clear how chemotherapy impacts on overall survival. Particularly for patients who have a low-grade oligodendroglioma or who have mixed oligoastrocytoma, chemotherapy may allow patients to defer radiation therapy for months or years.

In summary, despite the development of practice guidelines, it is still up to you and your doctor when you should undergo radiation therapy. You may also want to consider participation in a clinical trial studying new treatment approaches to the management of low-grade glioma.

44. Losing part of my hair during radiation therapy has been very hard for me. What can I do to make the experience more tolerable?

Hair loss in the area that received radiation is very common during radiation therapy. Hair loss from chemotherapy, on the other hand, affects hair all over the body. Being prepared for the loss of your hair will make the experience somewhat easier.

Typically, hair loss from chemotherapy or radiation is much easier for men, who may choose to "buzz it off" when it starts falling out. Women, on the other hand, have a more difficult time, and the thought of losing some or all of their hair is more personal.

Even before radiation or chemotherapy begins, many people look for a wig or hairpiece in the same color or style as their natural hair to ease the transition to hair loss. Some women have purchased several different style wigs and made a game of it: "Who will I be today?" Your doctor may write a prescription for a wig or hairpiece because the loss of your hair is associated with your cancer treatment. In fact, a wig in medical terminology is a "cranial prosthesis," referring to the protection that a hairpiece provides the scalp.

Your radiation oncologist will be able to tell you, based on your treatment plan, where you will lose your hair, since you will not lose all of it unless you have whole-brain radiation therapy. For example, you may be able to keep your hair longer on the top to cover areas of hair loss over the temporal lobes. Patients who lose hair over the front of the scalp may choose to wear a scarf or hat that covers only the bare areas. If you will lose a large portion of your hair or if you will have odd-shaped areas

Even before radiation or chemotherapy begins, many people look for a wig or hairpiece in the same color or style as their natural hair to ease the transition to hair loss.

Radiation Therapy

of hair loss, you may choose to cut your hair short to make it easier to cover with a hairpiece. Cutting your hair short before it starts to fall out makes it somewhat more manageable when it does begin to fall out. You can also use a mild shampoo and conditioner and avoid blow-drying it to help avoid irritating your scalp.

Scarves, turbans, hats, and other head coverings can also be used on the days when you prefer not to wear a hairpiece. The American Cancer Society publishes a catalog of wigs and various head coverings (www.tlcdirect.org). Many other websites specialize in hairpieces for chemotherapy-related hair loss (www.paulayoung.com, www.williamcollierdesign.com, and www.allusionshair.com). Also, many communities have a boutique designed for men and women who have hair loss related to cancer treatment.

M.L.'s comment:

Although the amount of hair loss that people have after radiation is variable, more than likely you'll lose at least some of it. I did, and it was very upsetting to see those first clumps of hair come out in the bathroom sink. The radiation therapist told me that on average most people start to experience hair loss around 2 weeks after the start of radiation treatments. I tried to prepare for it, but I still cried when it happened. You have to keep telling yourself it's all part of the healing process. I continued to remind myself that the radiation that was making my hair fall out was also continuing to eat away at those "bad cells" in my brain, and that was a good thing. I just tried to stay strong through all of it. I kept telling myself that my hair would grow back. I found that wearing a "doo rag" on my head with a baseball cap over it made me feel kind of cool. My husband has a motorcycle, and he took me to a shop where they sold motorcycles, clothing, and accessories. One of the accessories that motorcyclists wear when they are riding is a doo rag. It keeps the rider's hair from flying all over the place, and it makes the helmet a bit more comfortable. I found that a doo rag looked a lot better on me than a scarf or bandanna, so I started wearing them every day. It was funny when people started asking me where I had bought them.

Radiation Therapy

Chemotherapy and Other Drug Therapy

What is the blood–brain barrier? How does it determine which drugs are used in brain tumor treatment?

What are the most common chemotherapy drugs used to treat brain tumors? What are their side effects?

What can I do to prevent or diminish the side effects of chemotherapy?

More . . .

45. What is the blood–brain barrier? How does it determine which drugs are used in brain tumor treatment?

The tiny blood vessels or capillaries of the brain that deliver oxygen and nutrients to the cells differ from the capillaries of other organs. The walls of the capillaries of most of the body are porous so that molecules move freely from the bloodstream into the tissues. The walls of the capillaries of the brain, on the other hand, are more tightly joined together. This tight seam or "junction" restricts the movement of larger molecules, including drug molecules, into the brain. The **blood–brain barrier** refers to the limitation imposed on drugs and other substances from crossing the capillary walls into brain tissues (**Figure 20**).

Blood–brain barrier

Tightly joined cells in the blood vessels of the brain that prevent the ready diffusion of substances into the brain tissue.

Clearly, many drugs readily pass into the brain (e.g., alcohol, cocaine, and all types of "recreational" drugs!), but other drugs have physical characteristics that prevent their passage through the capillaries. Some brain tumors have more "leaky" capillaries and therefore do not have an intact blood–brain barrier. These tumors tend to show an area of bright contrast enhancement on an MRI (magnetic resonance imaging) scan when intravenous gadolinium has been used (see Question 17).

Some chemotherapy drugs, including carmustine (BCNU), lomustine (CCNU), temozolomide (Temodar), and procarbazine (Matulane), have the ability to cross the intact blood–brain barrier. The drugs cisplatin, carboplatin, and vincristine do not cross the intact blood–brain barrier well, but they may be effective in malignant tumors, which have capillaries that are more porous.

The significance of the blood–brain barrier in determining the success of chemotherapy in brain tumors

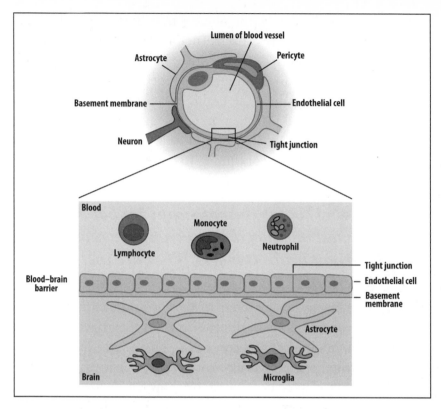

Figure 20   The blood–brain barrier.

Source: Reprinted with permission from Expert Reviews in Molecular Medicine, Cambridge University Press, 2003.

has been debated for many years. The presence of "leaky" capillaries within the tumor may allow the chemotherapy drug to kill more of the surrounding tumor cells. It is possible to open the blood–brain barrier temporarily with drugs such as mannitol. This process, called blood–brain barrier disruption, has been developed in some research centers as a way to achieve higher concentrations of chemotherapy to the tumor and to the surrounding brain tissues, which may contain scattered tumor cells. This has been particularly useful in treating primary central nervous system (CNS) lymphoma, which is a very chemotherapy-sensitive tumor.

Unfortunately, the blood–brain barrier does not prevent systemic cancers, such as breast cancer and lung cancer, from spreading into the brain and spinal fluid. It may, however, limit the penetration of chemotherapy drugs into the brain. For example, a lung cancer patient taking chemotherapy may have shrinkage of his lung cancer at the same time that metastases in the brain are continuing to grow.

46. What is chemotherapy? What are the most common chemotherapy drugs used to treat brain tumors? What are their side effects?

Chemotherapy refers to the medications used to treat cancer that have direct effects on the growth and proliferation of cancer cells.

Chemotherapy refers to the medications used to treat cancer that have direct effects on the growth and proliferation of cancer cells. There are hundreds of chemotherapy drugs, and they are divided into different classes depending on how they affect the cell. Most chemotherapy drugs interfere with the reproductive cycle of cancer cells by affecting their DNA, but some block other steps in cell division. Unfortunately, the effects of chemotherapy on some of the body's normal cells, particularly the rapidly dividing cells of the bone marrow, can cause considerable toxicity. Because the bone marrow produces red blood cells, white blood cells, and platelets, chemotherapy can kill these cells, sometimes placing the patient at risk for infection or bleeding.

Chemotherapy is usually given in cycles. Each cycle consists of the day or days in which chemotherapy is given and the time it takes for bone marrow to recover or other toxicity to resolve. The cycle length varies according to the drug or combination of drugs; it may be as short as 2 weeks or as long as 8 weeks.

It is difficult to list all of the drugs that have been used in the treatment of primary and metastatic tumors; however, some drugs have been developed specifically for the treatment of primary brain tumors. Others have shown effectiveness in clinical trials; some of these drugs are already approved by the **Food and Drug Administration** (FDA) to treat other conditions. These drugs may be considered off-label for use in the treatment of brain tumors (see Question 60). Some drugs are best known by their generic name and others by their trade name; the names used most commonly will be used for simplicity.

The drugs BCNU (carmustine) and CCNU (lomustine) are some of the oldest drugs used to treat astrocytomas, oligodendrogliomas, and many other types of brain tumors. BCNU is an intravenous drug, and its chemically related cousin, CCNU, is an oral drug. BCNU and CCNU have good penetration across the blood–brain barrier, but they may affect blood cell counts for several weeks; therefore, these drugs are commonly given in cycles 6 to 8 weeks apart. In addition to their effects on blood cell counts, these drugs can cause lung scarring (pulmonary fibrosis), a condition that may cause shortness of breath. BCNU and CCNU have been used in combination with other chemotherapy drugs. For example, CCNU is commonly used in combination with procarbazine and vincristine in a drug regimen known as PCV.

BCNU has been incorporated into a wafer, which is designed to dissolve in the brain when placed into the surgical cavity after tumor resection. The Gliadel wafer does not affect blood cell counts or cause lung toxicity, but it may not be used in patients whose tumors cannot be resected. When using Gliadel, the neurosurgeon

Chemotherapy and Other Drug Therapy

Food and Drug Administration (FDA)

A federal institution charged with approving and regulating medications, foodstuffs, and other products for human consumption.

must take precautions to make sure spinal fluid containing BCNU does not contaminate the surgical wound. Currently, Gliadel is approved to treat glioblastoma multiforme, although off-label use of the wafer has included patients with other resectable primary or metastatic tumors.

Temozolomide (Temodar) is an oral drug developed in Europe that was approved for treatment of recurrent anaplastic astrocytoma in the United States in 1999. Since that time, many other tumor types have been studied in clinical trials with Temodar. Some clinical trials have explored the use of Temodar in combination with other drugs and with radiation therapy. Many different administration schedules have also been used, but the most common schedule used in the United States prescribes that Temodar is taken daily, at bedtime, for 5 days, every 4 weeks. Lower doses of Temodar have been used daily during radiation or on protracted schedules after radiation. Most patients tolerate Temodar well without experiencing significant effects on blood counts. Temodar has not been shown to cause lung damage. It may cause nausea and constipation, but both can usually be controlled with other medications. Temodar does not cause hair loss, although in rare cases, it may cause a rash.

Recently, it has been shown that patients who have received Temodar on a 5-day schedule may have better tumor control with a longer, low-dose schedule. In some cases, up to 30% of patients who did not have tumor control with a 5-day schedule are successfully treated on a daily low-dose schedule.

Temodar is also available as an intravenous preparation, which is an advantage for patients who have difficulty swallowing.

Procarbazine (Matulane) is an oral chemotherapy drug that may be used alone or in combination with other chemotherapy drugs. This drug, however, interacts with other drugs, including antihistamines, narcotics, some nausea medications, and alcohol. Procarbazine can also cause high blood pressure when used in combination with foods high in tyramine, such as brewer's yeast, chicken liver, bananas, and aged cheese. A study comparing Temodar and procarbazine in recurrent glioblastoma found that Temodar causes less toxicity and appears to be more effective than procarbazine, although procarbazine is still widely used in combination therapy.

Methotrexate has been used primarily to treat CNS lymphoma. It is often given in high doses and is followed with administration of leucovorin, a drug that acts as an antidote for methotrexate toxicity in normal cells. High doses are necessary to penetrate into spinal fluid and treat leptomeningeal cancer cells.

Carboplatin and cisplatin are often used to treat lung cancer, ovarian cancer, and other malignancies. They have been used intravenously and intra-arterially in primary brain tumors. Cisplatin may cause kidney damage, peripheral neuropathy (numbness and tingling, particularly in the lower extremities), and severe nausea. Carboplatin has less severe nausea, but is more toxic to blood cells, especially platelets.

Cyclophosphamide (Cytoxan) is an intravenous drug that has been used for pediatric and adult brain tumors such as medulloblastoma. It causes low blood cell counts and nausea.

CPT-11 (Camptosar, also called irinotecan) is an intravenous drug that was originally approved to treat colon cancer. Clinical trials have shown that CPT-11 is effective in treating malignant glioma. Several different doses and schedules have been used. Recently, it has been used in combination with Avastin, a new targeted therapy (see Question 53).

Etoposide (VP-16) has been used orally and intravenously to treat many different types of cancer. It has been used in combination with other drugs to treat medulloblastoma, germinoma, and primitive neuroectodermal tumors. It has also been used to treat metastatic small cell lung cancer.

Vincristine (Oncovin) is rarely used as a single drug in the treatment of cancer, but it is often used in combination with other drugs because it does not affect blood cell counts; however, vincristine may cause numbness, weakness, constipation, impotence, and other significant side effects. This drug is given intravenously.

Many other chemotherapy drugs have been used alone or in combination with other drugs to treat primary and metastatic brain tumors. Your oncologist or oncology nurse will give you references and information regarding the possible side effects of the drugs recommended to you before you start treatment.

47. What can I do to prevent or diminish the side effects of chemotherapy?

Because many chemotherapy drugs interfere with cell division, the rapidly dividing cells of the bone marrow—the white cells, red cells, and platelets—are the "innocent bystanders" of the toxic effects of chemotherapy. Fortunately, blood cell counts usually recover rapidly, often within days, but some drugs have longer effects on the blood cell counts. Your doctor or nurse will explain to you which of your blood cell counts may be affected by your chemotherapy and what you should expect while your blood cell counts may be low. If your blood cell counts remain lower than expected, it may become necessary for your doctor to reduce the dosage of your chemotherapy.

White blood cells (**neutrophils, lymphocytes**, and **monocytes**) protect your body against infection. Neutrophils, also called segmented neutrophils or polymorphonuclear leukocytes, are the first line of defense against bacterial infections and fungal infections. These cells often multiply rapidly during the early stages of an infection. For example, a high white blood cell count may signal a serious infection such as pneumonia; however, if the patient is undergoing chemotherapy, the white blood cell count may be lower than usual—particularly, when the neutrophil count is very low (a condition called **neutropenia**), the patient is at more risk for severe infection. It is important to notify your doctor if you develop a fever, cough, or other symptoms of infection when your white cell count may be low. A number of different drugs, including sargramostim (Leukine), filgrastim (Neupogen), and pegfilgrastim (Neulasta), may be administered by injection to stimulate recovery of your neutrophil count to normal. In some situations, your doctor may need to hospitalize you to treat fever or infection while your white blood cell count is low.

The red blood cell count may also be affected by chemotherapy. A low red blood cell count (**anemia**) may result from a number of other causes, including iron deficiency. For this reason, you should be careful to include iron-rich foods in your diet while you are on chemotherapy. Anemia can cause fatigue and shortness

White blood cells (neutrophils, lymphocytes, and monocytes) protect your body against infection.

Neutrophil

Type of white blood cell.

Lymphocytes

Type of white blood cell found in lymphatic tissue such as lymph nodes, spleen, and bone marrow.

Monocytes

Type of white blood cells normally found in the lymph nodes, spleen, bone marrow, and within tissue.

Neutropenia

A lower than normal neutrophil count.

Anemia

Low red blood cell count; may cause tiredness, weakness, and shortness of breath.

Chemotherapy and Other Drug Therapy

of breath. In severe cases of anemia, it may be necessary to have a transfusion of red blood cells. Epoetin alfa (Procrit), an injectable red blood cell growth factor, may be recommended by your oncologist if your red blood cell count falls during chemotherapy.

Thrombocytopenia

Low platelet count.

Platelets are important in normal clotting, and a very low platelet count (**thrombocytopenia**) may be associated with severe bleeding. If necessary, a low platelet count can be treated with transfusion. Oprevelkin (Neumega) is an injectable drug that is used to stimulate the recovery of platelets. It is administered for several days after chemotherapy, when thrombocytopenia is anticipated.

Although nausea is a common side effect of chemotherapy, the widespread use of more effective antiemetic (antinausea) medications has significantly decreased the incidence of nausea and vomiting. Medications such as ondansetron (Zofran), granisetron (Kytril), and dolasetron (Anzemet), and a long-acting drug, palisetron (Aloxi), can be given intravenously or orally before chemotherapy. These drugs, unlike some of the older medications, do not cause sedation, making it safer for patients to receive chemotherapy in the outpatient setting. Most of the chemotherapy drugs used to treat brain tumors cause nausea; for this reason, oncologists recommend that patients receive **antiemetic medication** before taking chemotherapy rather than waiting to see if nausea will develop. It is particularly important to prevent vomiting when taking an oral chemotherapy drug because it cannot be "doubled up" if a dose is missed.

Antiemetic medications

Drugs that prevent nausea and vomiting.

Other side effects, including constipation, diarrhea, and fatigue, are quite variable from patient to patient and can also vary with the dose of the chemotherapy drug used. Your doctor or nurse will explain more about the side effects of each drug you will receive and the measures that you can take to avoid the side effects.

Another side effect often associated with chemotherapy is hair loss. Some of the more common chemotherapy drugs, such as Temodar, BCNU, CCNU, and carboplatin, do not cause hair loss; however, your oncologist will explain whether the drugs you will receive are associated with hair loss so that you can prepare for this (see Question 44).

M.L.'s comment:

I think the fear of nausea and vomiting is the most common concern with chemotherapy. It certainly was for me! I rarely experienced any sickness while I was on chemotherapy, and I could hardly believe it. I took Temodar for 23 months and had severe nausea only on the first night that I took it. I think I probably was so nervous about whether I would get sick that I probably brought the nausea and vomiting on myself. I'll never really know whether it was the drug or my nerves that made me sick, but I do know that I took the antinausea medication every single time that I took my Temodar, and it helped.

The side effect that I DID have was just a general feeling of being tired, but not so tired that I couldn't go to work. There were days that I would go home early or go in late. For the first couple of days that I was on chemotherapy, I was fine. I didn't feel tired at all; however, as the week went on and more chemotherapy was in my body, I started to become more tired. I remember wanting to sleep in later than usual, and I would fall asleep earlier in the evening than usual. This wasn't really a bad thing. I just felt like it was the reality. of being on chemo, and hey, it was a lot better than feeling nauseous.

Another side effect that I felt was loss of appetite. For me, that was a good thing because I had gained so much weight while I was on steroids that I wanted to lose some weight. In talking with others who were on Temodar, I found that the loss of appetite affects everyone differently. There were some people who said they didn't have much of an appetite for anything. Others, like me, only had a slight loss of appetite. The good news was that my normal appetite came back shortly after I finished each round of chemotherapy.

One other side effect that occurred while I was taking Temodar was constipation. If you've ever been really constipated, you know that it isn't something that you want to experience very often. I found that I didn't experience the constipation if I took a powdered laxative mixed in with orange juice once a day for every day that I was on chemotherapy. Most of the time, I would extend taking the laxative a few more days until I felt like the chemotherapy had gone through my system and my appetite was back to normal.

All in all, my experience with Temodar was surprisingly positive. I didn't get sick, and I didn't lose my hair. Yes, I was a little fatigued and my appetite was down, but this only lasted for about 5 to 7 days. Once I figured out how to address the constipation, that wasn't even an issue any more. In short, I'll take the fatigue, loss of appetite, and the constipation over NOT getting sick or losing my hair any day of the week!

48. I saw two oncologists after the diagnosis of my tumor, and both recommended chemotherapy for my tumor; however, one recommended taking a combination of chemotherapy drugs and the other recommended a single drug. Both seemed to have good reasons for their recommendations, but how do I decide who's right?

Your oncologist's choice of a treatment regimen involves many variables. Although some oncologists adhere to published guidelines or the "standard of care," others readily adopt new drugs or regimens as soon as there are published reports that a new therapy results in an improved outcome. Many treatment recommendations evolve from the results of clinical trials (see Part Seven), but such trials may take several years to complete.

An oncologist also takes into consideration your other medications, health problems, and any previous therapy you may have had. The cost of the treatment must also be considered, as some insurance companies will not cover drugs that are used "off-label" (see Question 60).

Even for relatively rare tumors, such as CNS lymphoma, a number of different chemotherapy drugs have proven successful in treatment. In many treatment protocols for CNS lymphoma, for example, high-dose methotrexate has been used, but there are many variations in the dose, the schedule, and even the duration of infusion; therefore, there is more than "one right answer," and your oncologist may have chosen the treatment with which she has had the most experience.

Oncologists may also differ in the number of cycles of chemotherapy they recommend. For most brain tumors, the optimal duration of chemotherapy treatment is not known. In the past, when drugs such as CCNU and BCNU were the mainstay of treatment, few patients could tolerate several months of therapy because of the development of toxicity to the bone marrow and lungs. Newer drugs such as Temodar are not as toxic, and many patients can tolerate treatment for a year or longer; however, if there is no evidence of residual tumor on an MRI after several months of treatment, it is still not clear whether patients should continue chemotherapy or continue follow-up without active treatment.

Fortunately, there is not just one "right" answer to questions regarding treatment. A number of treatment approaches have been developed over the past 10 years, and recommendations continue to evolve from the results of clinical trials. If you desire aggressive treatment because of the possibility of residual tumor, you should communicate this to your oncologist. It is also important to convey to your oncologist your expectations regarding your treatment so that you can openly discuss whether the two of you agree. Some physicians expect their patients to be partners in all decisions concerning treatment; others are less willing to be open to a patient's suggestions. This difference in style can be very critical as you proceed through treatment; thus, remember that your treatment may entail more than your initial chemotherapy regimen.

If you desire aggressive treatment because of the possibility of residual tumor, you should communicate this to your oncologist.

Finally, as with other issues regarding treatment, if you are considering participation in a clinical trial, you must make certain that you will keep your eligibility for the trial. Some clinical trials do not allow patients who have had chemotherapy to participate. Others will not allow patients to participate if they have received more than one or two drugs. If participating in a specific clinical trial is important to you, be sure to contact the center offering the trial before you begin another treatment.

49. Why are some drugs given orally, through a vein, or through an artery, whereas other drugs are delivered into the spinal fluid or into the tumor cavity?

All of the drugs commonly used in the treatment of cancer have been studied for several years in research animals and in clinical trials. During those studies, some drugs were noted to be easily absorbed through the gastrointestinal tract when taken orally, a characteristic called **bioavailability**; however, some drugs are not absorbed or lose their effectiveness when administered orally. These drugs have not been manufactured in an oral form and are only available as an injectable (usually intravenous) preparation. Temodar is an oral drug with good bioavailability; CPT-11 has poor bioavailability and is always given intravenously.

Relatively few drugs have been studied by directly injecting them into an artery that supplies the tumor (**intra-arterial administration**). Also, only a few drugs have been proven safe to inject directly into spinal fluid (**intrathecal administration**). In general, research centers that specialize in drug development use **animal models** to determine the safety and effectiveness of drugs to use by these special routes. The chemotherapy wafer Gliadel, which contains the drug BCNU, is currently the only chemotherapy approved for administration into the tumor cavity (**intracavitary administration**). At some centers, drugs have been administered through small catheters directly into

Bioavailability

Chemical property of a drug describing its absorption through the gastrointestinal tract when taken orally.

Intra-arterial administration

Injection into an artery that supplies blood to the tumor.

Intrathecal administration

The injection of a drug directly into the spinal fluid.

Animal models

Laboratory animals that have diseases similar to those in humans.

Intracavitary administration

The administration of a drug directly into the tumor cavity.

**Convection-
enhanced delivery**

Infusion of drugs into
the brain through
inserted catheters

the area surrounding the tumor, a technique called
convection-enhanced delivery.

50. I have had surgery, radiation therapy, and chemotherapy. My oncologist recently said that after a year of treatment I have had a "complete remission." I asked him whether this is the same as being cured; he said no. What is the difference between remission and cure?

Remission (from the Latin word *remissio*, to send
back) means that the symptoms of a disease and the
objective evidence of the disease have partially or completely resolved. A **partial remission** (PR) means that
some evidence of the tumor remains. In a clinical trial,
at least a 50% reduction in the original size of the
tumor must occur before a patient is considered in PR.
The complete resolution of all signs and symptoms of
disease is a **complete remission** (CR). Because of the
posttreatment abnormalities that may persist for several months on an MRI, it can be difficult to define
when a brain tumor patient achieves CR.

**Partial
remission (PR)**

Shrinkage or partial
disappearance of a
tumor, but with evi-
dence that some of
the tumor still exists.

**Complete
remission (CR)**

Complete resolution
of all signs and symp-
toms of disease.

Having a stable MRI scan for months or years does not
necessarily mean, however, that a patient is cured. Most
people would define cure as the permanent eradication of
disease. It would be impossible to verify over a period as
short as 12 months that the disease is permanently eradi-
cated. In the absence of effective treatment, microscopic
disease may eventually grow back into a visible tumor.

Although most patients want to know what their
chances are for a cure, the answer is never 100%, and it
is never 0%. The chance of achieving remission, however,
may be quite high. The next question typically asked is
this: "How long will the remission last?" Because of the

variation in growth rates among different types of brain tumors, this can also vary widely. For example, primary CNS lymphoma is a malignant tumor that may involve the brain and spinal fluid. If a patient completes treatment and the MRI of the brain shows no evidence of disease but the patient still has malignant cells in the spinal fluid, the patient's "response" to treatment would be considered a PR. A patient is considered a CR only when *all* evidence of disease has resolved with treatment. Some of those patients may be cured.

Because of the known risk of relapse, however, these patients are followed regularly for any recurrence of disease. In fact, a complete remission may last only a matter of weeks after discontinuing treatment.

It is important to understand that when using the word "remission" your doctor is not trying to avoid the word "cure." Your doctor is merely trying to describe as accurately as possible the presence or absence of disease.

51. My cancer was found in the spinal fluid. My doctor says that chemotherapy can be given directly into the spinal fluid with an Ommaya reservoir. What is an Ommaya reservoir, and how is it used for chemotherapy?

For patients who have cancer cells in the spinal fluid, or leptomeningeal spread, small doses of chemotherapy can be injected into the spinal fluid to circulate in the ventricles and over and around the spinal cord and spinal nerves. Although some patients receive chemotherapy injections with a spinal tap or lumbar puncture, this may be impractical or technically difficult for patients who require treatment for several months.

Chemotherapy and Other Drug Therapy

Ommaya reservoir

A hollow, slightly dome-shaped device is attached to a catheter that is surgically implanted into the cerebral ventricle. Chemotherapy is administered by injection into the reservoir and catheter.

An **Ommaya reservoir** is a hollow, slightly dome-shaped silicone device that is attached to a catheter, surgically implanted by a neurosurgeon in the operating room. The catheter is threaded though a small hole in the skull into the nondominant cerebral hemisphere, often the right frontal lobe. The hollow reservoir is slipped between the skin of the scalp and the skull. The slightly rounded surface of the reservoir allows your doctor to locate its placement, and the surface of the skin is cleansed with an antibacterial solution. A butterfly needle is inserted through the skin into the dome to "access" the reservoir. Spinal fluid is removed by slowly aspirating with a syringe, and chemotherapy is then administered by injecting it into the reservoir and catheter. Most patients have no discomfort when chemotherapy is administered through the Ommaya reservoir, and the procedure can be easily performed within minutes on an outpatient basis (**Figure 21**).

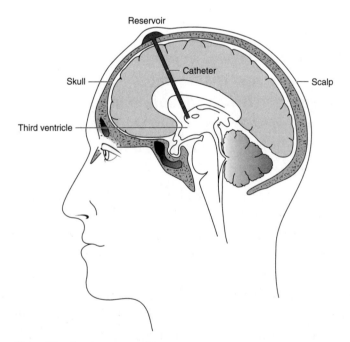

Figure 21   Ommaya reservoir.

Strict adherence to sterile techniques is essential when the reservoir is accessed because the introduction of infection into the spinal fluid can be life threatening. Fortunately, after the skin at the insertion site of the reservoir heals, no special precautions are required on the part of the patient.

Patients who have an Ommaya reservoir for chemotherapy may require lifelong reevaluation of the spinal fluid to detect evidence of recurrence. For this reason, the Ommaya reservoir is considered a permanent device. It is not removed at the end of treatment.

Table 4 lists drugs that have been used for intrathecal therapy. Methotrexate is by far the most common drug used in intrathecal therapy. DepoCyt, which was approved a few years ago, is specifically formulated to persist over time so that it requires less frequent injections. Newer drugs, such as topotecan, are still being studied in clinical trials to determine which tumors respond best. Your oncologist will provide further information about the drug and potential side effects before you begin treatment.

Table 4   Drugs Used in Intrathecal Therapy

Drug	Types of Cancer Treated
Methotrexate	Breast cancer, lymphoma, leukemia
Cytarabine (Ara-C)	Lymphoma, leukemia
DepoCyt (liposomal encapsulated cytarabine)	Leukemia, lymphoma
Thiotepa	Lymphoma, leukemia, breast cancer
Etopophos	Lymphoma, lung cancer, germinoma, glial tumors
Topotecan	Lymphoma, small cell lung cancer, glial tumors
Dacarbazine	Melanoma

Chemotherapy and Other Drug Therapy

Cancer cells in the spinal fluid may be very difficult to detect, as very few "float" in the spinal fluid even when a patient may have had symptoms for several months.

Cancer cells in the spinal fluid may be very difficult to detect, as very few "float" in the spinal fluid even when a patient may have had symptoms for several months. Even in patients with Ommaya reservoirs, a lumbar puncture may be necessary to sample the spinal fluid to make sure that cells are not persistent within the lumbar spinal fluid (as not all cells seem to circulate throughout the ventricles and spinal fluid pathways to the same degree). Also, some patients have numbness, tingling, or other sensory changes that may signal either a persistent tumor or side effects from intrathecal chemotherapy. Despite these concerns, treatment of leptomeningeal cancer can be well-tolerated, effective, and life saving.

52. Why should I have a different type of chemotherapy if the first type did not work?

There are many reasons why a particular chemotherapy drug may be ineffective in the treatment of a tumor. Many chemotherapy drugs have to be administered at a certain dose or schedule for maximum benefit, but the patient may not tolerate this dose. Sometimes the drug seems to work for several months; nevertheless, the tumor eventually begins to grow, possibly as a result of the development of drug resistance. Also, if one subpopulation of tumor cells was always resistant to the drug, the successful destruction of the sensitive cells will unmask this growing subpopulation.

Chemotherapy drugs that belong to different classes may have different success rates. In general, it is difficult—if not impossible—to predict at diagnosis which drug is best for a given patient. Several laboratories have developed testing procedures to determine the most effective drugs against a patient's tumor (**Figure 22**). The assay requires that a portion of the live tumor removed during surgery is submitted for analysis. Although the assay

Chemotherapy and Other Drug Therapy

ONCOTECH
15601 Red Hill Ave.
Tustin, California 92780
800-462-6832
714-566-0420
Fax: 714-566-0421
CLIA ID 05D0643386
CAP Cert. 37638-01

Patient Name:	XXXXXXXXX, XXXXX	Diagnosis:	Glioblastoma
Date of Birth:	XX/XX/XX	Prior Chemotherapy:	Yes
Oncotech ID No:	XXXXXXXXX	Specimen Site:	Brain
Institution:	XXXXXXXXXXXXXXX	Specimen Size:	1 GM
Oncologist:	XXXXXXXXXXXXXXX	Collection Date:	XX/XX/XXXX
Surgeon:	XXXXXXXXXXXXXXX	Date Received:	XX/X/XXXX
Pathologist:	XXXXXXXXXXXXXXX	Date Reported:	XX/X/XXXX
Medical Record:	XXXXXXXXXXXXXXX	Date Printed:	XX/X/XXXX
Pathology Ref. No:	XXXXXXX	Report Page No:	1

DRUG RESISTANCE ASSAY

TEST CODE 100

	ASSAY-PREDICTED RESPONSE PROBABILITY	Literature Response Rate
CISPLATIN	20	10
TEMOZOLOMIDE	14	10
DOXORUBICIN	13	10
VINCRISTINE	3	10
ETOPOSIDE	<3	5
CARMUSTINE	<3	10
CYCLOPHOSPHAMIDE	<3	10

Low Drug Resistance — Intermediate Drug Resistance — Extreme Drug Resistance

Sample Report

-1.0 | Median 1.0 | 2.0
Relative In Vitro Cell Proliferation

The graph above represents relative tumor cell proliferation observed in the presence of each drug tested. Longer bars indicate greater in vitro proliferation and therefore greater resistance to a particular drug. Literature response rate is determined from an extensive review of clinical trials. Assay predicted response probability derives from an algorithm involving in vitro tumor cell proliferation, literature response rate, and patient treatment status, in accordance with the Bayesian mathematical model.

The Oncotech EDR Assay is a drug resistance assay. Use of the Oncotech EDR Assay to identify and/or select clinically active agents is not recommended.

This test was developed and its performance characteristics determined by Oncotech, Inc. It has not been cleared or approved by the U.S. Food and Drug Administration. The FDA has determined that such clearance or approval is not necessary. This test is used for clinical purposes. It should not be regarded as investigational or for research. This laboratory is regulated under the Clinical Laboratory Improvement Amendments of 1988 (CLIA) as qualified to perform high complexity clinical testing.

Rev. 3-05

ONCOTECH
15601 Red Hill Ave.
Tustin, California 92780
800-462-6832
714-566-0420
Fax: 714-566-0421
CLIA ID 05D0643386
CAP Cert. 37638-01

Prognostic and Predictive Marker Report

Patient Name:	XXXXXXXXX, XXXX	Diagnosis:	Glioblastoma
Date of Birth:	XX/XX/XX	Prior Chemotherapy:	Yes
Oncotech ID No:	XXXXXXXXXXXXXXX	Specimen Site:	Brain
Institution:	XXXXXXXXXXXXXXX	Specimen Size:	1 GM
Oncologist:	XXXXXXXXXXXXXXX	Collection Date:	XX/XX/XXXX
Surgeon:	XXXXXXXXXXXXXXX	Date Received:	XX/X/XXXX
Pathologist:	XXXXXXXXXXXXXXX	Date Reported:	XX/X/XXXX
Medical Record:	XXXXXXXXXXXXXXX	Date Printed:	XX/X/XXXX
Pathology Ref. No:	XXXXXXX	Report Page No:	1

DNA Test Results and Histogram

Test Code	DNA Study	DNA Result	Favorable	Intermediate	Unfavorable
				Relative Risk Assessment	
400	DNA Ploidy	Aneuploid	Diploid	N/A	Aneuploid
	DNA Index	1.8	1.0	-	>1.0 or <1.0
	S-Phase Fraction	17.5%	See Note	See Note	See Note

NOTE: Percent S-phase fraction is associated with proliferative activity, however, the prognostic significance of the S-phase fraction in this tumor is still unknown at this time, and therefore, reference ranges are not available.

Aneuploid G0G1

Note: Green peak denotes Diploid G0/G1.

Interpretational Guidelines for DNA

Patients with aneuploid tumors have been shown to have a shorter disease-free survival period than patients with diploid tumors. Percent S-phase fraction is an additional prognostic marker and patients with elevated S-phase have increased probability of relapse. DNA content analysis has not yet been established as a diagnostic procedure and should be used only in conjunction with medically established tests and diagnostic procedures.

Test Results

Test Code	Marker	% Cells	Staining Intensity	Results / Histoscore	Favorable	Intermediate	Unfavorable
						Relative Risk Assessment	
500	HER2/neu	0%	0+	Not Detected	Not Detected	Not Established	Detected
520	p53 Gene Product	0%	0+	Not Detected	Not Detected	Not Established	Detected
540	Ki-67	70%		70%	<15%	NA	>15%
545	MGMT	20%	1+	Detected	Not Established	Not Established	Detected
580	Angiogenesis/CD31	30/200X field		See Comment	Not Established	Not Established	Not Established
	Comment: Reference range for malignancy of Glioblastomas has not been established. The process of new capillary formation in tumors is termed angiogenesis (neovascularization). The increase in blood supply facilitates the rapid growth of the tumor and provides an avenue for the escape and relocation of tumor cells to distant sites. A high degree of tumor angiogenesis has been associated with a shorter disease free survival in breast, prostate and other tumors.						
585	GST PI	80%	2+	Detected	Not Detected	Not Established	Detected
	GST-pi is a cytosolic enzyme which catalyzes the conjugation of toxic compounds to glutathione for transport out of the cell. Increased expression of GST-pi has been demonstrated to show increased resistance to alkylating agents such as cyclophosphamide, ifosphamide, and melphalan.						

These tests were developed and their performance characteristics determined by Oncotech, Inc. They have not been cleared or approved by the U.S. Food and Drug Administration. The FDA has determined that such clearance or approval is not necessary. These tests are used for clinical purposes. They should not be regarded as investigational or for research. This laboratory is regulated under the Clinical Laboratory Improvement Amendment of 1988 (CLIA) as qualified to perform high complexity testing.

Rev. 3-05

Figure 22   Sample reports from Oncotech, which includes chemosensitivity testing as well as other prognostic markers for glioblastoma.

takes several days, it may be possible to identify certain drugs that are more effective against the tumor; however, such testing cannot duplicate the many factors that affect the success or failure of a given therapy. The patient's immune system, the blood–brain barrier, and the blood supply to the tumor all affect the effectiveness of treatment delivered intravenously or orally. These factors cannot be duplicated in chemotherapy sensitivity assays. Also, there is a chance that the patient will develop intolerable side effects to the drug. For this reason, pretreatment predictive testing is not always helpful.

In some instances, a drug that is chemically distinct from the first drug used may be more effective. For example, it is known that brain tumor cells are sometimes resistant to the chemotherapy drug BCNU; therefore, tumor cells that are resistant to BCNU may also be resistant to CCNU because the drugs are closely related. The drug CPT-11, however, is from another class of drugs, and thus, tumor cells may not be resistant to this drug.

In an effort to develop treatment strategies that prevent the development of resistance, some centers have used sequential chemotherapy drugs in alternating cycles. If a tumor cell survived the first drug, it may not survive the second or third. Also, some researchers (and Dr. Ben Williams, a noted glioblastoma survivor and author) have developed combinations of drugs administered simultaneously. These approaches have resulted in long-term survival of some patients, although as of yet, the multiple-drug approach has not become the standard of care. Multiple-drug regimens have the advantage of confronting the heterogeneity of many brain tumors, possibly limiting the development of drug resistance; however, each drug may have separate or even additive toxicities.

Is there any hope of response—or cure—when a patient has already had three or four separate drugs without any apparent effect on the tumor? Yes. Because of the differences between drugs (and new drugs continue to be developed), some patients will have a successful outcome despite previous failures. Because of the previous treatments, however, the **bone marrow reserve** (see Question 62) may be limited, and that is why multiple treatment regimens may be more difficult for the patient to tolerate.

53. What is targeted therapy? Could targeted therapy be of benefit in treating my tumor?

Targeted therapy uses drugs or other substances such as monoclonal antibodies to identify and attack specific cancer cells without harming normal cells. It differs from chemotherapy in that the latter interferes with cell division and function; targeted therapies interfere with specific molecular cell-signaling pathways in cancer cells. Chemotherapy is typically given at the highest dose tolerated by normal cells (e.g., allowing significant but temporary effects on blood cells), but targeted therapy is dosed to inhibit a specific pathway, which may have no effect on blood counts at all.

Many older drugs could be considered targeted therapy, such as the hormone therapies used for breast cancer. The newer agents are not hormonal, however; they may target processes common to many types of cancer. Targeted therapies may even interfere with more than one signaling pathway at once.

Because there are so many molecular differences between brain tumor cells and normal cells, there are many potential molecular targets. Researchers study the entire cancer cell cycle, as well as invasion, blood vessel growth, metastasis, and drug resistance, to identify the signals that allow the cancer cells to grow and spread.

Bone marrow reserve

Term used by oncologists to describe the expectation of recovery of bone marrow cells after treatment with chemotherapy or radiation therapy.

Chemotherapy and Other Drug Therapy

One characteristic of cancer cells that has received much attention over the last several years is that of angiogenesis, the production of new blood vessels that allows a tumor to grow. Some brain tumors produce a protein called vascular endothelial growth factor (VEGF), which promotes rapid and extensive blood vessel growth. In fact, one of the characteristics that defines glioblastoma is its vascular proliferation.

Several drugs have been developed as targeted therapy against VEGF, and some have been studied extensively in brain tumors. Avastin (bevacizumab), a monoclonal antibody given by intravenous infusion, binds to

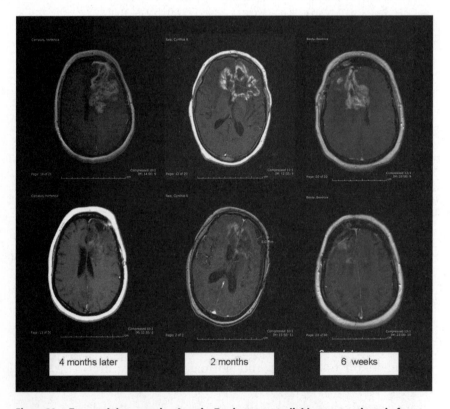

Figure 23 Targeted therapy using Avastin. Top images are glioblastoma patients before receiving Avastin; bottom images show the same patients and the length of time since starting treatment.

VEGF in the blood stream and prevents VEGF from reaching its target, the VEGF receptor. This "starves" the tumor and also reduces the edema or fluid accumulation around the tumor (Color Plate 7).

The first study with Avastin in patients with recurrent malignant gliomas, in combination with CPT-11, showed that an amazing 90% of patients had a complete response, partial response, or disease stabilization. Almost all patients had improvement in the edema surrounding the tumor, often resulting in neurological improvement within a few days after receiving therapy. Further studies with Avastin, as a single agent and in combination with multiple other chemotherapy and targeted therapies, have shown rapid improvement in glioblastoma and in other malignant brain tumors. Although many patients eventually have progression on Avastin, some have sustained complete remissions with little toxicity.

Avastin had been associated with CNS hemorrhage in another cancer metastatic to the brain, but the incidence of hemorrhage with Avastin in malignant gliomas appears to be very low. Its most significant side effect is its impact on wound healing, which also requires the development of new blood vessels; therefore, Avastin cannot be used for several weeks after surgery and should be avoided if surgery is planned. Rarely, patients have developed perforation of the bowel; in some cases, these patients had known gastrointestinal conditions that may have predisposed them to perforation. Avastin has been associated with high blood pressure, fatigue, and nosebleeds, but it does not affect blood counts. Avastin is the first **antiangiogenesis** therapy that has been approved for use in glioblastoma patients.

There are two other oral drugs, Nexavar (sorafenib) and Sutent (sunitinib), that also inhibit angiogenesis and

Antiangiogenesis

Property of a drug or other treatment that prevents the formation of new blood vessels.

that have been approved for use in kidney cancer. Both have been used in some brain tumor trials but do not appear to be as effective or as well tolerated as Avastin. **Figure 24** shows other new drugs and their targets.

Another targeted therapy, Tarceva (erotinib), is an oral drug that inhibits epidermal growth factor receptor (EGFR). This growth factor is associated with many cancers, including about one-third of glioblastomas. Although an early study showed little benefit when Tarceva was used alone, further studies with Tarceva combined with chemotherapy appear more promising. Tarceva and Avastin have also proven effective in

AKT
• Perifosine

Angiopoietin Inhibitors
• Amgen 386

Aurora Kinase Inhibitors

Chk kinase Inhibitors

EGFR
• Gefitinib (ZD1839, Iressa)
• Erlotinib (OSI-774, Tarceva)
• Lapatinib (GW-572016)
• AEE788
• ZD6474
• BIBW 2992

Farnesyltransferase
• Tipifarnib (R115777, Zarnestra)
• Lonafarnib (Sch66336, Sarasar)

HGF
• Amgen 102

Hif-1α

Histone Deacetylase
• Depsipeptide
• Suberoylanilide hydroxamic acid (SAHA)

Hsp90 Inhibitors
• IPI-504
• XL888
• SNX5422
• CUDC 305

IGFR

Integrins
• Cilengitide (EMD 121974)
• M200

mTOR
• Temsirolimis (CCI 779)
• Everolimus (RAD 001)
• Rapamycin (Sirolimus)
• AP23573

PDGF
• Gleevec (imatinib mesylate)
• PTK787
• SU101
• SUO11248
• GW786034
• MLN518

PI3K
• BEZ225

PKC
• Tamoxifen

PKC β2
• Enzastaurin (LY317615)

PLK Inhbitors

Proteosome
• Bortezomib (Velcade)

RAF kinase
• Sorafenib (Bay 43-9006)

Src
• Sprycel (Dasatinib)

TGF-β/TGF-β Receptor
• SB-431542
• AP12009

VEGF/VEGFR
• Avastin (Bevacizumab)
• Angiocept (CT-322)
• Sorafenib (Bay 43-9006)
• Semaxanib (SU5416)
• VEGF-TRAP
• PTK787
• SU011248
• AEE788
• AZD2171
• ZD6474
• AMG 706
• GW786034
• CEP-7055

2^{23} = 8,388,608 possible combinatorial pairs across the major categories

SNO: 2008

Figure 24   Targeted molecular agents: A partial list of cellular targets and the corresponding drugs used.

Source: Dr. David Reardon, Duke University.

combination, with 92% of patients achieving response or stable disease.

Zactima (vandetanib) is an oral drug that is effective against both VEGF and EGFR. In early studies, Zactima was associated with disease regression or stability in half of the patients treated and seemed to be well-tolerated.

Gleevec (imatinib) was developed for chronic myelogenous leukemia but has been shown to also inhibit platelet derived growth factor (PDGF). Some glioblastomas test positive for the PDGF receptor and are sensitive to Gleevec. This is more common when a low-grade glioma has transformed over time to the more malignant glioblastoma (see Question 1). Gleevec has had limited success when used alone but is currently being used in combination with other agents.

Cilengitide (EMD 121974) is an intravenous drug that seems to have antiangiogenesis effects and limits the spread of tumor cells within the brain. It appears to have very little toxicity, and in studies combining cilengitide with standard radiation and Temodar in newly diagnosed glioblastoma patients, its addition appeared to improve survival compared with radiation and Temodar alone.

It should be clear from the previous discussion that many targeted therapies have shown promise in the treatment of brain tumors, and new drugs and combinations continue to be studied. Because of the low toxicity of many of these agents, patients may feel better, with less risk of severe infection or anemia. Many of the targeted therapies have been FDA–approved for diseases other than brain tumors and may be denied insurance coverage; however, it is important to discuss this with your oncologist, as some pharmaceutical companies have programs to underwrite the cost of the drugs.

54. I have been hearing about brain tumor vaccines. What are they, and when will they be available?

Most people think of a vaccine as an injection given to prevent a disease such as smallpox, measles, tetanus, or other infection. Currently, only one vaccine is available to prevent cancer, the human papillomavirus vaccine, given to prevent cervical cancer. Brain tumor vaccines, like many other cancer vaccines, are given to patients diagnosed with the disease to prevent recurrence.

Currently, only one vaccine is available to prevent cancer, the human papillomavirus vaccine, given to prevent cervical cancer.

Several vaccines have been developed over the last few years at cancer centers across the country, and a vaccine commercially available in Switzerland, DCVax-Brain, is in clinical trials in the United States. The DCVax product is made by combining the patient's own dendritic cells, a type of white blood cell that directs an immune response against foreign proteins on the tumor cells. Some of the patient's tumor cells from a brain biopsy are cultured with the dendritic cells to "train" the dendritic cells to recognize them. The dendritic cells are then administered by a series of injections.

Another vaccine, called Oncophage, also made from the patient's own tumor, has shown promising results in recurrent glioblastoma. A similar vaccine is being developed for melanoma and kidney cancer.

Celldex Therapeutics has developed a vaccine that uses a synthetic version of a mutant EGFR protein. For patients whose tumors express the EGFR protein variant III (EGFRvIII), the vaccine stimulates two arms of the immune system, T and B cells, to attack the tumor.

This vaccine could potentially be used in any patients whose tumor expressed the EGFRvIII protein, without having to remove a portion of the tumor to culture.

In most of the studies thus far, vaccines have been used in patients with relatively small tumors, often in combination with Temodar. Ideally, vaccines would be administered after the initial surgery, when the number of residual tumor cells is low and the patient's immune system has not been adversely affected by other cancer treatments. It appears that most of the vaccines have little if any toxicity. Dr. Keith Black, one of the developers of the dendritic cell vaccine, anticipates that cancer vaccines may be directly injected into recurrent tumors, avoiding the risk of more invasive surgery.

Like all new therapies, vaccines must be evaluated and approved by the FDA before they will be commercially available in the United States; however, the rapid accrual to the vaccine clinical trials predicts that the studies will be completed in the near future and may be available within the next year.

55. What other drugs could be used to treat my tumor?

A number of different drugs have been used to treat malignant brain tumors, some alone and some in combination with chemotherapy. The majority of clinical trials to determine the effectiveness of these drugs have been conducted in patients with malignant glioma, and thus, less is known about their usefulness in the treatment of other types of brain tumors.

Accutane (13-cis-retinoic acid) is an oral drug that has been approved for the treatment of cystic acne. It is known that some malignant gliomas have an epidermal growth factor receptor that, when chemically blocked, prevents cell division. Accutane appears to block the epidermal growth factor receptor. Clinical trials have shown that some patients are long-term survivors when given high-dose Accutane therapy. Accutane has also been used in combination with Temodar, improving survival over Temodar alone. Although Accutane has shown to improve survival, it does have side effects, including dry skin and lips, headache, and nausea. It can also cause birth defects.

Thalidomide (Thalomid), another oral drug, is believed to inhibit growth of tumor cells by interfering with the tumor's ability to grow new blood vessels (antiangiogenesis). Thalidomide was developed as a sedative in Europe but was associated with devastating birth defects. It did not receive FDA approval until it was shown to be effective in treating leprosy. Thalidomide is effective in the treatment of a blood disorder, multiple myeloma, and has also been used in clinical trials for patients with malignant glioma. Used alone, it seems to slow the growth of tumors, although some patients experience tumor regression. Thalidomide has been used in combination with Temodar, CPT-11, and carboplatin. Its major side effects, sedation and constipation, are usually manageable. Both male and female patients are required to practice effective contraception while taking thalidomide.

Other commercially available drugs that may inhibit angiogenesis include the cyclooxygenase-2 inhibitor Celebrex, which is typically used to treat arthritis. In addition to treating arthritis, these drugs have shown to inhibit tumor growth in animal models. Both drugs have been used in the treatment of cancer, alone and in combination with chemotherapy. Side effects include nausea, headache, and stomach ulcers.

Tamoxifen (Nolvadex) has been used for several years in the treatment of breast cancer. When administered in higher doses, this drug has shown to be effective in the treatment of malignant glioma. It is believed that at higher doses tamoxifen inhibits a cell-signaling enzyme called protein kinase C, which prevents glioma cell division. Doses of tamoxifen used for treating brain tumor patients are 10 to 12 times higher than those commonly used for treating breast cancer. High doses of tamoxifen may be associated with **deep vein thrombosis** (DVT), the formation of blood clots in the extremities (see Question 67). It may also cause nausea, hot flashes, and weight gain. A recent study suggested that patients on high-dose tamoxifen had an improvement in survival when first treated with medication to reduce thyroid hormone production.

Deep vein thrombosis (DVT)
Blood clot forming in deep veins, often with impaired or sluggish blood flow.

An antimalarial drug, chloroquine, has been added to chemotherapy in low doses to prevent drug resistance. Although not used extensively in the United States, chloroquine has attracted attention because of studies in Mexico that showed an impressive improvement in survival, even in patients with large tumors, who received chloroquine concurrently with chemotherapy.

A number of other nonchemotherapy drugs are in clinical trials. Because many are considerably less toxic than chemotherapy, new combinations of nonchemotherapy drugs and standard chemotherapy regimens appear promising.

A number of other nonchemotherapy drugs are in clinical trials.

It should be apparent from the previous descriptions that hundreds of clinical trials with different combinations of agents are possible. Although traditionally most brain tumor clinical trials in the United States have studied one or two agents at a time, Dr. Henry Friedman of Duke University has urged neuro-oncologists to embrace multiagent therapy, using the most effective agents together or in sequence. Dr. Ben Williams, a glioblastoma survivor since 1995, has written extensively on the topic of drug cocktails, using both pharmaceutical agents and nutritional supplements to target multiple growth pathways concurrently.

56. How long should I stay on treatment?

The duration of treatment depends on many factors, but ultimately, it depends on your response to treatment and the toxicity that you experience while on treatment. Patients on clinical trials may have a specific duration of therapy planned as part of the trial or may continue therapy as long as their tumor appears to be responding. Some oncologists stop treatment after the tumor has been in remission for at least 2 months, but it is often difficult to determine whether there is an active tumor remaining. Preliminary studies indicate that patients with malignant glioma who continue Temodar for longer than 1 year have an improvement in overall survival.

Nitrosoureas such as BCNU and CCNU have cumulative toxicity, sometimes causing prolonged periods of low blood counts as treatment continues. Both drugs may also be associated with lung scarring (pulmonary fibrosis), which may be irreversible. These drugs are rarely given for a year or more for this reason. Temodar, Procarbazine, and CPT-11 have been given for longer periods without significant cumulative toxicity, but almost all chemotherapy drugs affect the blood cell counts and may require a reduction in dose if they are continued. Also, drugs such as Accutane, thalidomide, and tamoxifen may be taken without significant long-term toxicity, but no one knows the optimal duration of therapy.

57. Are all types of chemotherapy for brain tumors covered by insurance?

Private insurance, Medicare, and Medicaid may pay for some types of chemotherapy but not for others. For example, intravenous drugs such as BCNU may be covered by all three providers. Temodar is covered for primary brain tumors by most private insurers, and Medicare covers some but not all of the cost. Off-label use of drugs (drugs approved for one type of tumor but not specifically approved for brain tumors, see Question 60) may not be covered by Medicare or Medicaid. Even some private insurers may not cover a drug that is considered "experimental." Check with your doctor or your insurance company if you are unsure about whether your chemotherapy is covered.

If you are interested in a drug that is not covered on your insurance, you may be able to receive the drug through a pharmaceutical company program. Some programs are open to patients without drug coverage, and some are open to any patient denied access to a drug by their insurance company. Websites such as www.NeedyMeds.com and www.Xubex.com list prescription drugs that are available from the manufacturer.

PART SEVEN

Clinical Trials for Brain Tumor Patients

What is a clinical trial?

What do I need to know before I enroll in a study?

What is the difference between an investigational therapy, an "off-label" drug, a complementary therapy, and an alternative therapy?

More . . .

58. My doctor told me that I'm "a perfect candidate for a clinical trial," but I'm not sure what he means by this. What is a clinical trial?

A clinical trial is a study of patients with similar characteristics designed to answer a specific question or set of questions. Ideally, clinical trials study small populations, but they are intended to yield answers that may be applied to a larger population of similar patients. A clinical trial may study people who have not had a disease but are at risk for developing it. A clinical trial may test the effectiveness of a new drug or study a different way to give an older drug. A clinical trial may ask patients to give blood samples or tissue samples for testing after receiving different doses of a drug. A clinical trial may compare two different types of therapy in two sets of patients to determine which treatment is better tolerated or more effective. At least two components are common to all clinical trials: (1) a written research plan, or **protocol**, written for the investigators conducting the study, and (2) the informed consent, which tells the patient what the clinical trial is designed to do and what the patient is expected to do as part of the study.

Protocol

A research plan for how a therapy is given and to whom it is given.

As in these examples, not all clinical trials are designed to test new therapies. Although many new drugs or treatment strategies have been studied in a clinical trial, many questions are unanswered because no clinical trial has yet studied them.

If your doctor has encouraged you to find out more about clinical trials and said that you are a "perfect candidate," he is not only paying you a compliment—he is also telling you something about your medical condition. A patient who enters a clinical trial must be able to understand the principles of the trial he is considering.

This does not mean that the patient needs a college degree, but it does mean that the patient should not have unrealistic expectations about the purpose of the trial and what the clinical trial will do for him as an individual. Clinical trials are not written for the benefit of individual patients; they are written to further the development of new treatments for a future population of patients. Also, patients who have severe medical problems that may interfere with the treatment on the trial are not eligible to participate in the study.

Clinical trials may be offered by your physician if he is associated with a university, research center, pharmaceutical company, or other institution. Some clinical trials are "multicenter" trials and are offered at multiple institutions around the country or internationally. Some clinical trials are very small, enrolling less than 50 patients. Others enroll hundreds of patients and may take years to complete.

Clinical trials may be offered by your physician if he is associated with a university, research center, pharmaceutical company, or other institution.

Many universities, regional cancer centers, and community cancer programs participate in clinical trials. Pharmaceutical companies sponsor some clinical trials, private foundations sponsor others, and still others are sponsored by the National Cancer Institute (NCI). The NCI provides financial support to cancer centers around the United States that participate in clinical research organizations, such as New Approaches to Brain Tumor Therapy (NABTT), the Southwest Oncology Group (SWOG), and the Eastern Cooperative Oncology Group (ECOG). In addition, NCI conducts clinical trials at the National Institutes of Health (NIH) Clinical Center in Bethesda, Maryland. Clinical trials that are supported by NCI can be located on the Internet at: www.cancer.gov/clinical_trials. In addition, many individual cancer centers have websites that list their current clinical trials (see Question 100). Finally, Dr. Al Musella's web portal www.virtualtrials.com contains a comprehensive listing of clinical trials for brain tumor patients.

59. I'm interested in finding a clinical trial of a new treatment for glioblastoma multiforme. What do I need to know before I enroll in a study?

Patients who are interested in enrolling in a clinical trial should be commended! Participation in a clinical trial can be time consuming, inconvenient, and expensive, and patients are not paid for their participation. Some clinical trials may require frequent visits to a clinic or research center. Some trials may require more frequent testing than traditional therapy outside of a clinical trial. Some trials may require surgery or other invasive procedures; however, the only accurate way to answer questions about the side effects and effectiveness of new therapies is with a carefully conducted clinical trial.

Pilot study

Small study designed to test an idea or treatment prior to a larger clinical trial; also called a feasibility study.

Sponsor

The organization that funds a research study or clinical trial.

Several different types of clinical trials are available. A **pilot study** or feasibility study is a small study of a new therapy or technology that may be very complicated or expensive. This type of study involves a small group of patients. It allows investigators to determine whether a larger trial should be performed. In some cases, the **sponsor** of a study (the organization that funds the research) will require that the new therapy show promise before allowing a large number of patients to receive it. An example of a pilot study is a trial that studies a group of brain tumor patients who are on the same therapy at 2-month intervals using magnetic resonance imaging (MRI), positron emission tomography (PET), and a new imaging modality. The purpose of the study is to determine whether the new imaging technique provides additional information that may help predict the patient's response to therapy.

Preclinical studies are studies that use live animals to determine whether a particular treatment affects the heart, lungs, kidneys, and other organs. Animal models (animals with implanted tumors) are given the treatment to determine whether the treatment kills tumors without harming the animals. Other animal studies are conducted in normal animals to determine the effects of large doses of a drug. This type of study reveals the possible side effects that a human will experience after several months of taking the drug.

Sample Preclinical Trial

Suppose that a new drug, YZ-1234, is discovered to kill human brain tumor cells in cell cultures. When administered to laboratory mice that have been implanted with human brain tumors, the tumors appear to shrink. YZ-1234 is then administered in larger doses to normal animals to determine its side effects. If any of the animals die after receiving the large doses of YZ-1234, their organs are studied to determine why they died. The results of these studies determine whether the drug is considered safe and effective enough to test in human subjects. In this example, some of the information is derived from cell cultures. In this way, multiple types of cells can be studied: brain tumor cells, breast cancer cells, lung cancer cells, and so forth. Also, because many cell lines grow quickly in cultures, these studies can be performed rapidly. Studies in cell lines, however, do not suggest whether the treatment will affect the kidneys, liver, heart, or other organs. For this reason, animal testing is required to ensure that the drug is safe before it can be tried in humans.

The Next Step

Phase I trial

Study of a small group of patients to determine the effectiveness and the side effects of a new treatment.

A **phase I trial** usually studies a small group of patients to determine whether a new treatment is safe, as the dose of the drug is gradually increased. Patients participating in a phase I study may not have the same type of tumor. In some cases, phase I studies are researching drugs that have not yet been studied in humans and the investigators begin the trial using a fraction of the dose found to be toxic in animals. The dose of the drug is gradually escalated in a small group of patients, with a careful review of side effects and laboratory tests. The next group of patients is given a slightly larger dose, and the toxicities are again reviewed. Dose escalations are repeated, sometimes several times, but when side effects of the drug are noted more frequently or become more severe, the trial is stopped. The side effect that is most severe is called the "dose-limiting toxicity" or DLT; for many chemotherapy drugs, the dose-limiting toxicities are low white cells, red cells, or platelets.

Pharmacokinetics

Study of how the body breaks down a drug after it is administered.

Blood and urine tests are obtained during treatment to determine how the dose of the drug given correlates with the level of the drug in the blood and how rapidly the body excretes it. These studies, called **pharmacokinetics**, are very important in determining how toxic the drug may be in different patients and whether the drug can be used in patients who are taking other drugs.

Phase I trials rarely result in successful control of the patient's tumor. Even when the drug has been very effective in animal studies, the dose that can be tolerated in humans may not kill the tumor. Although phase I studies do include diagnostic tests to determine whether the tumor has responded, the purpose of the study is to evaluate the *safety* of the drug, not its effectiveness.

If a patient decides to enter a phase I clinical trial, it is reasonable to ask whether "intrapatient dose escalation" is allowed. This refers to the practice of allowing the initial patients to receive a higher dose of the drug if they tolerate it well. For some drugs, receiving a higher dose increases the likelihood that the drug will be effective against the tumor.

Phase I clinical trials are usually open to patients of all tumor types and often allow patients who have had multiple other therapies. On the other hand, the risk of unforeseen toxicities and the relatively low likelihood of response are potential disadvantages of participation in this type of trial.

Sample Clinical Trial: Phase I

Back to our hypothetical new drug, which passed through preclinical studies: The next step is a phase I clinical trial. Patients entering this phase I clinical trial of the drug YZ-1234 receive one-tenth of the dose found to be toxic in mice. A small number of patients receiving YZ-1234 at the initial dose have no side effects, and thus, the next group of patients receiving YZ-1234 receives a slightly higher dose. The trial continues until the patients receiving YZ-1234 show abnormalities in their blood tests or side effects that the investigators determine to be toxic (the DLT) but reversible. The YZ-1234 dose that the investigators find to be tolerable is 200 mg per day.

Phase II Trials

A **phase II trial** studies a small group of patients, sometimes as few as 14, to determine whether there is a statistical likelihood that a new treatment will be

Phase II trial

Study of a group of similar patients to determine whether there is a statistical likelihood that a new treatment will be effective against a tumor.

effective against a specific type of tumor. Typically, the dose that was determined to be safe from the phase I trial will be used in all of the patients participating in the phase II trial. To determine whether the treatment is effective, it is important that all of the patients entered on a phase II trial are similar. The investigators usually set **exclusion criteria**, which may limit the patient's number of previous treatments before entering the study. Most phase II studies require that the patient have measurable disease because there must be a reference for determining whether the tumor is growing, shrinking, or remaining stable. If the new treatment appears promising in a proportion of the initial patients, the study may be expanded to allow more patients to receive the drug.

Exclusion criteria

Characteristics specified in a clinical trial that render the patient ineligible for the study.

Sample Clinical Trial: Phase II

In a phase II trial of YZ-1234, the drug is given to 14 glioblastoma patients who have previously had surgery and radiation therapy and have evidence of tumor recurrence after radiation therapy. These patients receive 200 mg of YZ-1234 per day. After 2 months of treatment, 3 patients have evidence of tumor response (shrinkage), 7 have no change, and 4 have evidence of tumor growth.

The Final Test: Phase III

A **phase III trial** compares two or more kinds of treatment in two or more similar groups of patients. Some phase III trials compare a new treatment that appeared promising in a phase II trial with the more standard therapy. Most phase III studies are randomized trials, meaning that the patients entering the trial are not given a choice of therapy. Instead, they are asked to

Phase III trial

Compares two or more kinds of treatment in two or more similar groups of patients, with one group of patients receiving the standard, or control, therapy.

accept a random chance of receiving either therapy. It is not known by either the investigators or the patients which arm of the trial contains the most effective therapy, although one arm may be less convenient, less toxic, or less expensive; therefore, it is very important to determine whether there is a definite survival benefit in one arm over the other.

Some phase III trials are **placebo** controlled, which would appear to be unfair to patients who are randomized to this group. A placebo often has the same appearance as the "real drug": the placebo may be a "sugar pill" of the same size and color or an intravenous solution of sugar water. Some placebo-controlled trials offer the same effective therapy in both arms of the trial, with the new drug or placebo added to detect whether there is any additional benefit. This also allows investigators to determine whether there are subtle side effects of the new therapy. For example, a placebo-controlled trial tested the Gliadel wafer, which contains the chemotherapy drug carmustine, in one-half of the patients having surgery for glioblastoma. The other glioblastoma patients also had surgery and had a placebo wafer implanted that was identical in appearance to Gliadel. Neither the patients nor their surgeons knew which patients were receiving which wafers because all treatment was coded. At the end of the study, the investigators matched the patients with the treatment they received and determined that, on average, the patients who received Gliadel lived longer. This finding was very important to determine with a placebo-controlled study because all patients had some benefit just by removing the tumor. Also, it was important to determine whether any side effects experienced by patients were related to the presence of the polymer wafer, even if it did not contain any chemotherapy.

Clinical Trials for Brain Tumor Patients

Placebo

A medication ("sugar pill") or treatment that has no effect on the body, often used in experimental studies to determine if the experimental medication/treatment has an effect.

Phase III studies are the largest, most time consuming, and most expensive clinical trials to conduct. They often require hundreds of patients to detect statistical benefit. Many phase III studies involve multiple research centers and take several years to complete. Phase III studies may have an interim analysis, which is designed to detect differences in the two groups before the study has been completed. An interim analysis may suggest such a striking difference in the expected outcome of the patients in the two arms that the investigators decide to stop the study early to avoid continuing to treat patients in the least effective way.

Sample Clinical Trial: Phase III

The new drug YZ-1234 appears to be less toxic and at least as effective as some of the previous treatments that have been used in glioblastoma; therefore, a phase III study of 500 glioblastoma patients is planned. In this study, 250 of the patients will be randomized to receive radiation therapy followed by YZ-1234. The other 250 patients will receive radiation therapy followed by Temodar, which was chosen because it is also an oral drug. It is estimated that the study will take 2 to 3 years to complete, and the study will be available at multiple centers to allow rapid accrual.

Deciding to Join a Trial

Patients who are considering enrollment in a clinical trial should understand that clinical trials involve an element of risk. These risks are explained in the informed consent document. The patient should never sign an informed consent if he does not understand the question being posed in the clinical trial.

Often the study title contains the phase of the trial and the names of any drugs or treatments being used. For example, the title for the phase I clinical trial discussed previously here would be as follows: "A Phase I Study of YZ-1234 in Patients with Advanced Cancer." The known side effects of the therapy proposed in the clinical trial must be carefully stated in the informed consent. The informed consent usually states that unusual or unforeseen side effects may also occur. The treatment alternatives, including the standard treatments for the disease, must be stated. The investigators must also disclose whether enrollment in the clinical trial would affect the patient's enrollment in future clinical trials. Most clinical trials state that effective contraception must be practiced during treatment in a clinical trial because of a possible risk to an unborn child.

Enrollment in a clinical trial may be restricted to patients who are "minimally pretreated" because certain drugs may be more toxic to patients who have already had different types of chemotherapy. For this reason, if you are considering participation in a clinical trial, it is important to consider this early in treatment.

60. What is the difference between an investigational therapy, an "off-label" drug, a complementary therapy, and an alternative therapy?

Investigational therapies or investigational drugs are treatments that are considered experimental or under development in a clinical trial setting. Some investigational drugs have not yet been approved for the treatment of any disease and cannot be obtained outside a clinical trial. Drugs that have been approved by the Food and Drug Administration (FDA) for the treatment of

Investigational therapies or investigational drugs are treatments that are considered experimental or under development in a clinical trial setting.

Investigational

Treatments that are experimental or under development in clinical trials, including drugs that were approved for other uses.

one type of cancer may be considered investigational for the treatment of another type of cancer. Also, drugs that may be approved for intravenous use may be considered investigational when used by another route, such as intra-arterially (injected directly into the artery supplying the tumor) or intrathecally (injected into the spinal fluid). Patients receiving investigational drugs on a clinical trial are allowed to continue taking the drug only if the treatment appears to be effective, as assessed by physical examination and diagnostic tests. An investigational drug may be supplied free of charge to a patient who is enrolled in a clinical trial; however, it is not always free, and the informed consent will specify this.

Off-label drug

A drug that is approved by the FDA for one type of treatment but may be prescribed for other conditions.

An **off-label drug** is approved by the FDA for one type of treatment but may be prescribed for other conditions. Some drugs may be both investigational and off-label; for example, the drug YZ-1234 may have been FDA-approved for colon cancer (a so-called labeled indication) but may be investigational and off-label for glioblastoma. Because of the time required and the expense of performing clinical trials, only a small fraction of research studies are performed solely to obtain FDA approval for a drug. Some drugs that are widely accepted in brain tumor therapy, such as procarbazine and vincristine, have not been FDA approved for this use. When clinical trials are published demonstrating that a treatment is effective and well-tolerated, doctors are more likely to prescribe the drug off-label. In some cases, insurance coverage does not reimburse for off-label use of the drug even when the patient's doctor determines that the drug is likely to be beneficial. You should always check with your doctor if you are concerned about whether your insurance will cover the drug.

Complementary therapies and alternative therapies encompass a variety of treatments, including herbal preparations, vitamin- or nutritional-based regimens, and therapeutic touch. **Complementary therapies** are used *in conjunction with* conventional therapy such as surgery, radiation therapy, and chemotherapy. **Alternative therapies** are used *in place of* conventional therapy. Some alternative therapies are based on the traditional medicines of other cultures, and others were developed by individual practitioners. A few alternative therapies have been studied in clinical trials. If you are interested in an alternative therapy, ask your doctor whether the treatment has been studied. It is also important to ask how long the treatment is expected to last because some alternative regimens cost hundreds or thousands of dollars a month. It has been estimated that up to 75% of all cancer patients use complementary therapy or alternative therapy at some point during their illness.

Although investigational therapy and alternative therapy are both options for the patient who does not want conventional therapy, there are many differences between the two approaches. Doctors who offer the patient investigational therapy judge the patient's response to treatment by conventional means such as neurological examination and MRI. Patients enrolled in a clinical trial for an investigational therapy may be asked to forego all other treatments (including alternative therapies) that may interfere with the therapy being studied.

Alternative therapies may be prescribed by naturopaths or herbalists who are not licensed to practice medicine, and therefore, they cannot order radiographic studies to determine response to treatment.

Complementary therapy

Treatment used in conjunction with standard treatment for disease.

Alternative therapy

Treatment used in lieu of standard medical therapies.

Clinical Trials for Brain Tumor Patients

Some naturopathic practitioners follow the principle of complementary therapy. They allow chemotherapy or radiation treatment at the same time as the alternative therapy. Many insurance plans do not cover the costs of alternative therapy, even when it has been prescribed by a licensed physician.

61. I am interested in a clinical trial at a research center in another state, but my doctor is opposed to this. He wants me to enter a trial at the medical school in my city or to take standard chemotherapy. What should I do?

There are many reasons that doctors do not refer their patients to clinical trials. If you have a good relationship with your local doctor and that doctor does not want you to participate in a particular clinical trial, make sure that you ask for the reasons. If you are not happy with your doctor's answer, it is certainly possible to change doctors to find one who is more accepting of the clinical trial you want. Although it is possible to enter a clinical trial in another state without a referral from your doctor, you still need to have a local doctor in case of an emergency. Do not assume that you will not need a local physician! You certainly do not want to have serious bleeding as a result of a low platelet count, for example, and be hundreds of miles from anyone who can arrange a platelet transfusion.

Some doctors are concerned that their patients assume that a clinical trial is better than standard therapy, but they know that the trial may not be successful. By definition, a new drug is being studied in a clinical trial because it has *not* proven superior to standard therapy. Moreover, less is known about a new drug than one that has already been studied and FDA approved. This is especially true when the clinical trial is a phase I study.

Some research centers have well-known doctors, famous patients, or new treatments that have received national media attention; however, in most clinical trials, only a few patients have the degree of success that is featured in the media. Your local doctor may be concerned that you are choosing a research center based on its reputation rather than its ability to offer you an appropriate treatment.

Some research centers manage the patient's care by having close communication with the local physician, and some do not. If the investigators running a clinical trial do not provide information about the investigational drug's side effects to a patient's local doctor, the local doctor is left "out of the loop." This may cause problems if the patient develops life-threatening complications related to the investigational drug, and the local physician has not been given any information about the side effects expected. If the patient comes to his hometown emergency room, the local doctor, not the research center doctor, will be called to see the patient. It is hardly surprising that the local physician will be unlikely to refer patients to that center in the future!

Some doctors feel that nearby medical schools should be supported in their research programs, and they may be more familiar with the investigators and the clinical trials offered at the local medical school. Your local doctor may also feel that frequent travel out of state will be more physically taxing on you than you realize.

It is best to schedule an appointment with your doctor to discuss your concerns. If you are considering conventional therapy after completion of the clinical trial, it is important to stay in touch with your local physician. Some outstanding brain tumor research programs, such as Duke University Medical Center, the University of California in San Francisco, and the University of California in Los Angeles, are very well regarded for their reputation in keeping local physicians informed of the patient's treatment.

62. I have received three separate chemotherapy drugs, and each seemed to work for several months. I now have an area of new tumor on my MRI scan. I'm interested in a clinical trial, but several of the clinical trials I have seen don't allow patients who have had previous chemotherapy to participate. Why is this?

Clinical trials enroll patients who are very similar—to level the playing field, so to speak. In a phase II clinical trial, in which the objective of the trial is to test the effectiveness of a new drug, patients who have had no chemotherapy at all often respond better than patients who have had multiple types of chemotherapy. Investigators have a better chance of evaluating the promise of a new drug if patients who are "heavily pretreated" are not enrolled.

Often an objective of the clinical trial is to determine the potential side effects of a new treatment. When selecting participants for this type of trial, a patient's bone marrow reserve is an important factor. Bone marrow reserve is the term that oncologists use to describe the expected recovery of the bone marrow cells—the cells that develop into the white blood cells, red blood cells, and platelets. This reserve is depleted when patients have had multiple treatment cycles of some chemotherapy drugs (particularly BCNU and CCNU). A patient whose bone marrow has been depleted by previous chemotherapy may require platelet transfusions or growth factors such as Neupogen after every subsequent chemotherapy cycle to help the blood counts return to a normal level. If that patient is included in a clinical trial designed to study the side effects of a new treatment, the new drug may decrease blood cell counts to very low levels. The patient may require dose reductions of the new drug to continue chemotherapy, which may then lessen the chances that the new drug will be effective.

Very healthy patients with good bone marrow reserve, normal kidney function, and normal liver function are the favored subjects for clinical trial investigators who are hoping that a highly successful drug can be rapidly approved for general use. Again, it is important to remember that clinical trials are not written to benefit individual patients. They are written to develop new therapeutic strategies.

63. I have heard a lot about herbal remedies, antioxidants, and other nontoxic treatments, but I was told that these treatments have not been studied in a clinical trial. Is this true? If it is true, why haven't these treatments been studied?

There has been an explosion of interest in so-called nontoxic therapies. Patients interested in such therapy can now investigate them and participate in clinical trials at a number of sites. The National Institutes of Health's National Center for Complementary and Alternative Medicine reports that an estimated $27 billion is spent on alternative and complementary therapies, such as herbal supplements, vitamins, plant extracts, shark cartilage, and hundreds of others. Some, but not all, supplements have been studied. Reviews of the results of these trials are now available.

Dr. Stephen Tomasovic, professor of molecular and cellular oncology at the MD Anderson Cancer Center, has compiled a list of complementary and alternative therapies and reviews of the scientific data, including the results of animal studies and clinical trials. This information is available on the web at: www.mdanderson.org/departments/CIMER. The list includes traditional Chinese medicine, herbal and plant therapies, biologic agents, special diets, and energy therapies. In addition, the site contains information regarding drug interactions, a glossary of terms, and a "Frequently Asked Questions" section.

In the past, researchers who were interested in studying herbal supplements or nontraditional therapy had difficulty attracting funding for animal studies and clinical trials. There are now a number of sources of funding for such trials, including research grants through the National Institutes of Health. Patients who are interested in clinical trials for complementary and alternative therapies must be willing to forego other treatments while on the clinical trial to avoid confusing the results of the study.

M.L.'s comment:

Early on, my husband read about clinical trials on the Internet. Further research has indicated to us that clinical trials are a very good thing. Participation in a clinical trial was never offered to me, but I understand that my tumor, anaplastic oligodendroglioma, isn't as common, and there were no clinical trials in my area for newly diagnosed tumors. Because the majority of my tumor had been resected through surgery, I wouldn't have been eligible for phase II clinical trials. These trials require a visible tumor to be present on a patient's MRI. My tumor responded so well to radiation therapy and chemotherapy that I still don't have enough visible tumor to qualify for a clinical trial . . . but this is fine by me! As I have continued to learn more about clinical trials over the years, I would like to offer a few words of caution. First, a location that has the term "research center" attached to it does NOT translate to "better" treatment. When speaking with brain tumor patients and/or their families, I have noticed on several occasions that this is something that they believe. It is important for you to know that this is not the case and that at times people can be misled simply because a particular center has a name that is well recognized by the general public or has the term "research center" attached to it.

Second, I have found that many brain tumor patients and families think that a clinical trial is better than standard treatment therapy. Again, this is not true. As a matter of fact, at the time of writing this update, I am a 9-year brain tumor survivor. I did not take part in a clinical trial, nor was I treated at a "well-known" research center. With that said, I did receive the best treatment available during the time of my treatment therapy (2000–2002).

One last point that I want to make about clinical trials is the importance of making sure that you keep your local physician informed about your treatments and the decisions that are being made. During your clinical trial, decisions may be made about your therapy, and if your local doctor(s) are not up to date with your changes, then a number of issues could arise—for example, certain side effects that need to be treated immediately (for example, a platelet transfusion) may not be as easily addressed as one might think.

PART EIGHT

Complications of Brain Tumors and Their Treatment

Can I expect to have brain damage as a result of surgery, radiation therapy, or other treatment?

I experience short periods in which I can't speak. This happens several times a day. I never black out, but my neurologist says that I could be having seizures. Is this common?

How long do I need to take anticonvulsant medication?

More . . .

64. Can I expect to have brain damage as a result of surgery, radiation therapy, or other treatment?

A neurological deficit (a change in the brain that results in abnormal or reduced function) does not necessarily follow surgery or other therapy. The size and the location of your tumor may actually be creating a neurological deficit. This may improve when the tumor is removed and the pressure on the nearby brain structures returns to normal.

Neurosurgeons carefully evaluate the tumor's position in relationship to the other brain structures. The type of surgery recommended is based on whether a permanent neurological deficit can be prevented. It is possible, however, that the tumor will be more difficult to remove than anticipated or that bleeding or other complications will occur after surgery. The neurosurgeon will explain all of these risks to you before surgery.

The temporary disability that may occur after surgery, which often improves with rehabilitation, must be distinguished from the late effects of radiation therapy and chemotherapy. Although loss of strength or coordination is upsetting to some patients, intellectual decline and loss of short-term memory can be even more devastating. These effects on cognitive function may occur in patients who have achieved remission; therefore, clinical trials that study these effects must separate patients who have cognitive loss because of tumor progression.

Most studies of cognitive decline after brain tumor treatment have occurred in children. These children were long-term survivors (5 years or longer), and most had received surgery and radiation therapy. Children who were younger at the time of diagnosis, who had larger radiation fields, and who had increased intracranial pressure at the time of diagnosis were found to be at an increased risk for IQ loss and poor performance in school.

In one study of adults who survived primary and metastatic brain tumors for at least 1 year; 12% suffered dementia and another 6% suffered psychological problems related to radiation therapy. Another study of adults treated for malignant brain tumors revealed that younger patients were more likely to improve over time, and most patients were able to return to their previous employment.

Patients at high risk for cognitive decline include those who are very young or very old at the time of diagnosis and treatment, those who have tumors of the cerebral hemispheres, and those who have radiation doses that include large daily fractions.

Although chemotherapy can also cause cognitive decline, it is sometimes difficult to separate the effects of chemotherapy from those caused by radiation therapy in patients who have received both types of treatment. For example, long-term survivors of primary central nervous system (CNS) lymphoma have a higher rate of cognitive decline with chemotherapy and whole-brain radiation therapy. High-dose chemotherapy paired with blood–brain barrier disruption, however, has not resulted in substantial intellectual impairment. This treatment success has increased the number of long-term survivors of primary CNS lymphoma, and thus, recent research has focused on maintaining intellectual function in patients. As a result, a number of treatment protocols for CNS lymphoma have eliminated whole-brain radiation therapy.

Although chemotherapy can also cause cognitive decline, it is sometimes difficult to separate the effects of chemotherapy from those caused by radiation therapy in patients who have received both types of treatment.

Prevention of long-term toxicity from radiation therapy is an area of active research. Your radiation oncologist may be able to advise you on available strategies that may reduce the risk of future complications.

M.L.'s comment:

My husband and my parents were concerned that I would come out of brain surgery a changed person. When a person goes into the operating room for other types of surgery, he or she comes out physically changed, meaning that the person may not have a bladder any more or may no longer have a breast. The person's emotional state may be temporarily unstable, but the mind remains the same. When a person undergoes surgery on the brain, there is a fear that the person who comes out of the surgery won't be the same person who went in. Your brain controls all of your functions, such as memory, speech, and motor skills. If a tumor is in a location near any of these functional areas, there is a very good chance that you may not have the same essence that you once had. The thought that "you don't come out the way you went in" is every patient and caregiver's concern.

65. I experience short periods in which I can't speak. This happens several times a day. I never black out, but my neurologist says that I could be having seizures. Is this common?

About one-third of all brain tumor patients have seizures. These seizures may occur as the first symptom or may occur months or years after diagnosis of a brain tumor. Some tumor types are more commonly associated with seizures, particularly oligodendrogliomas. Also, some areas of the brain, such as the temporal lobe, are more prone to seizures (**Figure 25**).

Seizures can be classified as partial or generalized. **Partial seizures** originate from a specific area in the brain, often the area around the tumor. A partial seizure

Partial seizure

Seizure involving only one area or lobe of the brain.

Types of Seizures	Characteristics/Symptoms
Partial Seizures	
• Simple Partial Seizures	Sometimes a precursor to complex partial seizure; no loss of consciousness; generally localized in one region of brain and involving one of these types of symptoms: • Somatosensory: tingling of contralateral limb, face, or side of body • Visual: sees flashes of light, scotomas, unilateral or bilateral blurring • Auditory: hears ringing, hissing, or noises • Autonomic: sweating, flushing or pallor, and/or epigastric sensations • Contraversive: head and eyes turned to opposite side • Focal motor: tonic–clonic movements or upper (or lower) limb
• Complex Partial Seizures	Similar to a simple partial seizure, but spreads to involve more than one area of the brain; patient may experience some of the symptoms associated with a simple partial seizure, then lose consciousness
Generalized Seizures	**Loss of consciousness; involves both brain hemispheres**
• Absence Seizures	Common in children; brief, vacant stare; eyes roll upward; eyelids flutter; cessation of activity; lack of response
• Myoclonic Seizures	One or several sudden muscle jerks, often while falling asleep or within a short time of waking up; can occur alone or with other generalized seizures

• Generalized Tonic–Clonic Seizures	1. Tonic phase:
	    Incontinence
	    Epileptic cry
	    Cyanosis
	    Generalized stiffening of body and limbs, back arched
	2. Clonic phase:
	    Cyanosis
	    Eyes blinking
	    Salivary frothing
	    Clonic jerks of limbs, body, and head
	3. Postictal confusional fatigue:
	    Limbs and body limp

• Atonic Seizures ("drop attack")	Sudden loss of muscle tone; head, neck, or whole body may drop; may include brief loss of consciousness

Figure 25 Types of seizures.

may have motor symptoms such as hand movement or sensory symptoms such as numbness or tingling. A simple partial seizure does not impair consciousness; a complex partial seizure does impair consciousness and the patient does not remember it.

Generalized seizures involve both cerebral hemispheres and impair consciousness. A tonic–clonic seizure, formerly called grand mal seizure, involves spasm of the body, limbs, and trunk muscles, and the patient may have difficulty breathing. The patient loses consciousness during the seizure and may be confused after the seizure. Weakness, muscle pain, and headache commonly occur after a tonic–clonic seizure.

Generalized seizure

Seizure involving both hemispheres of the brain.

179

Status epilepticus

A condition in which the patient has repeated seizures or a seizure prolonged for at least 30 minutes.

Status epilepticus, the continuation of a seizure or series of seizures without regaining consciousness, is a life-threatening condition. Patients with status epilepticus should be treated in an intensive care unit with intravenous medication and supplemental oxygen.

Electroencephalogram (EEG)

A recording of the electrical impulses of the brain using electrodes attached to the scalp.

An **electroencephalogram** (EEG) may be helpful in determining whether the episodes you experience are seizures; however, a normal EEG does not completely eliminate the possibility of a seizure disorder. In some hospitals, 24-hour EEG monitoring is available to determine whether a patient has infrequent seizures that may not be detected with a standard EEG.

It is important to tell your doctor of any seizures and to note whether seizures are becoming more frequent or more severe. Your doctor can often prescribe medication to lessen the frequency and severity of seizures.

66. I had seizures before my tumor was diagnosed, but I haven't had one since. How long do I need to take anticonvulsant medication?

Certain types of tumors are more commonly associated with seizures. These include lower-grade tumors such as oligodendroglioma, astrocytoma, ganglioglioma, and dysembryoplastic neuroepithelial tumors. Occasionally, gross total resection of the tumor is possible, and only short-term therapy with anticonvulsants is required, as long as the patient has remained seizure-free after the operation. Some patients can have surgical removal of both the tumor and an adjacent area that is determined during the operation to be the origin of the seizures. This may also allow eventual discontinuation of anticonvulsant therapy; however, your doctor will carefully review your situation before making any changes in your anticonvulsant therapy.

For patients with a residual tumor on an MRI (magnetic resonance imaging) scan, anticonvulsant therapy is often continued. Tumor progression, drug interactions, and electrolyte imbalances can trigger further seizures, even when anticonvulsant drugs are used. It is extremely important to comply with your doctor's recommendations regarding anticonvulsant medication and follow-up. Never taper or discontinue your anticonvulsant medication without checking with your doctor.

It is important to take your anticonvulsant medication consistently. Also, severe physical or emotional stress, alcohol, low blood sugar, and extreme fatigue can increase the risk of seizures. Your doctor may also prescribe "rescue" medications such as the Klonopin wafer or liquid Ativan that can be used in an emergency to stop a seizure.

M.L.'s comment:

As mentioned previously, while vacationing with my family in July 2008, I found out the hard way that someone can have a seizure after 9 years of remission! With absolutely no warning whatsoever, I experienced 3 grand mal seizures and ended up in the ICU for 3 days. With my initial diagnosis in 2000, I never knew for certain whether I had experienced a seizure in my sleep so my neurologist had recommended that I take anticonvulsant medication indefinitely. While I wasn't thrilled about this recommendation, I continued to take the medication. I took it for about 3 or 4 years, and in all that time, I never had a seizure. Occasionally, I asked my doctors whether I could stop my anticonvulsant meds (Keppra) altogether because I hadn't had a seizure. Some doctors said that I could wean off Keppra; others were against it. So, of course, I listened to the ones who said I could stop it!

As one would imagine, the seizures I experienced in 2008 were very frightening for my husband and I, as nothing like that had ever happened before. The doctor there did an MRI scan, which was normal, but I started back on Keppra. I still don't know why, after 9 years, I had the seizures, but I can only assume it was the fatigue from staying up late for several nights in a row and being out of my regular routine that may have contributed to it.

Once I got back home, I went back to see my doctors and told them everything that had happened. I had another MRI scan and an EEG, which were both normal. Within a week or so, I had my strength back and felt completely back to normal, but I took a few weeks off before I went back to work.

In Texas, one isn't allowed to drive for 6 months after a seizure. That was probably the worst thing about having a seizure. I'm just thankful that I didn't have one while driving.

67. Over the past several days, I have noticed that my left leg seems swollen and tight compared with my right. When I called my oncologist's office and talked to the nurse, she told me to go to the emergency room immediately. What's the problem? Why do I have to go to the emergency room?

The nurse is concerned that you may have a deep vein thrombosis (DVT), a blood clot in a large vein. The large veins of the legs may develop long, thick clots that block the return of blood flow to the heart. This can cause pain and swelling. The most dangerous complication of DVT, however, occurs if the clot breaks away from the walls of the vein and travels to the heart. A large clot can become lodged in the heart valves, but more commonly, the clot becomes lodged in the arteries of the lung. A clot that has clogged the pulmonary arteries is called a **pulmonary embolus**. A pulmonary embolus can cause sudden death. It has been estimated that up to 15% of all cancer patients die of pulmonary embolus.

Although DVT does not always result in pulmonary embolus, the presence of a clot in the extremities should be taken very seriously. Doctors hospitalize patients with DVT to keep them on bed rest, to begin anticoagulant therapy, and to evaluate for further evidence of pulmonary embolus.

A DVT in the lower limbs can be detected by ultrasound, which can detect blood flow through the veins below the surface of the skin and muscle. The most dangerous clots are those in the deep veins of the thigh and pelvis because these vessels are quite large.

A pulmonary embolus does not always cause symptoms. Some clots break up gradually, releasing a shower of small clots that lodge in the pulmonary vessels. A large clot typically causes shortness of breath, chest pain, or a cough. Although a chest X-ray may be normal, other tests, such as a ventilation/ perfusion scan or a chest computed tomography (CT) angiogram, may show a loss of normal blood flow to one or both lungs. Patients may require supplemental oxygen for several days because of this blockage of blood flow to the lung.

The most dangerous complication of DVT, however, occurs if the clot breaks away from the walls of the vein and travels to the heart.

Pulmonary embolus

Blood clot that travels through the veins and the heart, eventually occluding one or more pulmonary arteries.

Anticoagulants (blood thinners), such as heparin, enoxaparin (Lovenox), dalteparin (Fragmin), tinzaparin (Innohep), and fondaparinux (Arixtra), prevent the development of further clots; however, these drugs are all given by injection. Many patients prefer to take an oral anticoagulant called warfarin (Coumadin). Patients taking warfarin must be closely monitored with regular blood tests because of the drug's interactions with other medications and certain foods.

Some DVT patients, including those with recent neurosurgery, are at risk for bleeding complications from anticoagulants. Such patients may benefit from the placement of an **inferior vena cava (IVC) filter**, which is an internal device that is placed into the large vein below the heart to act as a screen for blood clots that may break off and travel to the heart and lungs. An inferior vena cava filter is often used in combination with an anticoagulant because DVT may still form in the limbs, causing pain and swelling (**Figure 26**).

It is not always possible to predict or prevent DVT. Patients who are not ambulatory, who have had recent

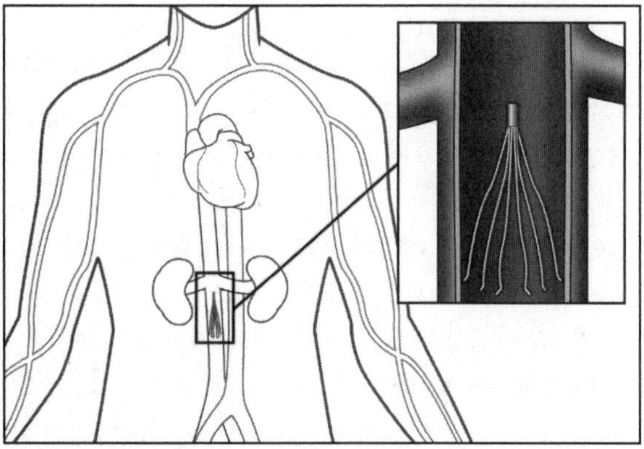

Inferior vena cava (IVC) filter

A vascular filter that is implanted into the inferior vena cava to prevent blood clots in the bloodstream from reaching the heart.

Figure 26   Inferior vena cava filter.

surgery, and who have a history of DVT should discuss ways to reduce the risk of DVT and pulmonary embolus with their doctors. Some doctors always prescribe a blood thinner if the patient is expected to be immobile for a long period of time, even if the patient has not had a previous history of blood clots.

68. Are infections more common in patients with brain tumors?

Brain tumor patients are not necessarily more susceptible to infection as a result of the tumor; however, their treatment may place them at risk for certain kinds of infections. Many brain tumor patients are treated with steroids such as dexamethasone before and after surgery. A short course of steroids usually does not increase the risk of infection; however, long-term steroid use (over a period of weeks or months) is often associated with fungal infections, particularly oral thrush (candidiasis). Thrush appears as a white coating over the tongue and back of the throat, and although it may be painless, it can affect taste and appetite. Extensive candidiasis of the esophagus and genitourinary tract may be painful and require several days of oral antifungal therapy.

Some chemotherapy drugs, especially when used in combination with steroids, increase the risk of infection. Temodar, a drug that is usually not associated with a low white blood cell count, affects the subset of white cells called lymphocytes that are important in preventing fungal and viral infections. Serious lung infections, including Pneumocystis, Aspergillus, and Nocardia, are rare in the normal population but are life threatening in patients with low lymphocyte counts.

Patients who have a history of herpes infections may also experience an increase in the number and severity of outbreaks.

Patients who develop a low neutrophil count (see Question 47) as a result of chemotherapy must take precautions to avoid infection and notify their doctors immediately for fever, chest congestion, or cough.

Patients who have implanted intravenous catheters for administering chemotherapy are at risk for infection and should notify their doctor if they experience any tenderness around the catheter or if they develop fever or chills.

Shingles, or herpes zoster, is a serious viral infection that often begins as a painful, tingling cluster of red blisters that rapidly become more extensive along the course of a nerve. Because of the pain associated with an outbreak of shingles, it is important to treat this infection as soon as possible. Even with treatment, the affected nerves can be painful for months or years after an outbreak.

69. Will my cancer treatments cause permanent infertility?

A number of different chemotherapy drugs can cause premature menopause, irregular menstrual periods, and infertility in women. Chemotherapy drugs can also cause infertility in men. Procarbazine, Temodar, cisplatin, and carboplatin have been associated with sterility. For some patients, the sterility is only temporary, and fertility is recovered within a year after stopping treatment; however, permanent sterility is more common in men and in women who are older than 40 years at the time of treatment.

Brain radiation can decrease or destroy the normal production of hormones that affect sexual development and reproduction. Men may benefit from testosterone injections to improve libido, decrease hot flashes, and prevent osteoporosis. Similarly, women who experience premature menopause after radiation therapy may benefit from low-dose estrogen and progesterone replacement therapy. Such therapy is usually prescribed to alleviate symptoms rather than to restore fertility.

Male patients who desire to father children after treatment may be able to bank sperm before starting therapy. For female patients, preservation and harvesting of eggs require considerably more time and expense. The need to initiate therapy as soon as possible may not provide enough time to retrieve viable eggs.

Some patients with pituitary tumors or tumors in areas near the pituitary gland may have abnormal sex hormone production at diagnosis. Disrupted hormone production may cause ovarian or testicular failure, resulting in infertility. Therefore, these patients cannot benefit from fertility preservation strategies before chemotherapy.

M.L.'s comment:

Several years after my radiation and chemotherapy treatments when I was about 41, I began to experience hot flashes and what I thought might be premature menopause. I asked my gynecologist about this and whether he thought this was related to my chemotherapy treatments. I also asked him if my chemo treatments could cause me to be infertile. He indicated that the hot flashes were more than likely related to my cancer treatments, but he also performed some tests to check my hormone levels. The results revealed that I was not infertile, which was very

Brain radiation can decrease or destroy the normal production of hormones that affect sexual development and reproduction.

Complications of Brain Tumors and Their Treatment

surprising, and I was thrilled. My gynecologist also pre-scribed me a hormone replacement medication called Pre-marin. I took it for a while, and it helped with the hot flashes; however, it also caused me to gain weight. So I talked to a nutritionist to find out if there was something else I could take that was more natural versus a medica-tion. Ground flax seed was recommended, and I have been taking it for about a year. It works great, but be sure to continue to take it or the hot flashes will come back.

70. I've always been healthy, but now that I have a brain tumor I worry about every little symptom. What symptoms should I look for, and when should I call my doctor?

It is not always easy to know when to call your doctor or even which doctor to call. Some problems can wait until your doctor can see you in the outpatient clinic, and some need immediate attention. At night or on the weekend, your doctor may direct you to the emergency room to check an X-ray, blood test, or culture. Make sure that you follow your doctor's recommendations.

If you have just had surgery, your neurosurgeon will want you to report any changes in your condition after you are discharged from the hospital. If you experience an infection in the surgical wound, a fever higher than 100°F, a sudden onset of a headache, or increasing weakness, call your neurosurgeon.

If you are seeing a neurologist for seizures, this doctor will manage your anticonvulsant medication and moni-tor any laboratory tests that might be required. Do not expect your other doctors to adjust your anticonvulsant medications. Your neurologist is expected to take charge in this area and will make any medication adjustments.

Your radiation oncologist will typically see you at least once a week during your treatment. After therapy is completed, most radiation oncologists will release you back to the care of your neurosurgeon, oncologist, or neurologist. If you develop a complication that requires admission to a hospital while you are receiving radiation therapy, let your radiation oncologist know. It may be possible to continue your treatment while hospitalized.

In many communities, a **medical oncologist** or neuro-oncologist assumes the care of a brain tumor patient after surgery. The medical oncologist or neuro-oncologist will work with the other specialists and your primary care doctor to arrange any laboratory tests or radiographic studies that you need. Although your primary care doctor may still treat other medical problems unrelated to the tumor (such as high blood pressure and diabetes), your oncologist will address the treatment of the brain tumor and any complications related to the tumor.

On the other hand, for some situations, you should not call your oncologist in the middle of the night. For example, a refill on your cholesterol medication, the results of an MRI scan taken earlier in the day, or a question about chemotherapy you received last month are not considered emergencies. Keep in mind that your doctor (or the partner who may be on call) will not have access to this information after office hours.

Make sure that you keep a card with all of your doctors' names and phone numbers available in your wallet in the event that another doctor needs to contact one of them regarding your care. It is also a good idea to have your pharmacy number and a 24-hour pharmacy number available in case your doctor needs to call in a prescription. **Table 5** lists common symptoms experienced

Medical oncologist

A physician who performs comprehensive management of cancer patients throughout all phases of care; specializes in treating cancer with medicine.

Complications of Brain Tumors and Their Treatment

Table 5 Problems to Report to your Oncologist

Problem	Possible Causes/Concerns
Sudden shortness of breath or chest pain	Pulmonary embolus or heart attack
Fever of 100°F or higher, especially when accompanied by chills	Severe infection
Swelling in one or both legs	Deep vein thrombosis
Severe nausea and vomiting or diarrhea	Could result in dehydration
Sudden onset of severe headache	Brain hemorrhage
Vomiting brown fluid or blood	Bleeding ulcer
Seizures that rapidly recur over a period of minutes	Onset of status epilepticus
Severe rash, especially one that involves the mouth or rectum	Life-threatening drug reaction
Numerous tiny red spots over the legs, bleeding gums	Low platelet count

by brain tumor patients that need to be reported to their doctor.

M.L.'s comment:

I used to think that the emergency room was just for life or death situations, but this is not the case. There is only so much your doctor can do for you over the phone or in the middle of the night when their offices are closed and staff/ nurses are not available.

I know that emergency rooms are probably the last place on earth you'd want to be when you're very ill. Most are very busy, and it can take hours to find out anything or get help for why you're there!

My advice would be to follow your doctor's instructions, and if he tells you to go to the emergency room, then you should go. They are open 24/7 and will be able to help you until your doctor is able to respond.

PART NINE

Medications Used in Brain Tumor Treatment

What does dexamethasone do? What are the side effects of dexamethasone?

What are the side effects of anticonvulsant medication?

My pharmacist said that there may be a "drug interaction" between some of my medications. What does this mean?

More . . .

71. After surgery, I was prescribed dexamethasone. My doctor says that I may be on this drug for several days. What does dexamethasone do? What are the side effects of dexamethasone?

Dexamethasone (Decadron) is a corticosteroid, a medication that reduces edema (swelling) around brain tumors by decreasing the tendency of fluid to leak from the blood vessels into the surrounding brain tissue.

Dexamethasone (Decadron) is a **corticosteroid**, a medication that reduces edema (swelling) around brain tumors by decreasing the tendency of fluid to leak from the blood vessels into the surrounding brain tissue. In addition to its effects in reducing edema, it is often used with chemotherapy to control nausea and vomiting. Dexamethasone is available as an intravenous form or in tablets.

Most brain tumor patients are given dexamethasone before surgery, and many have noticed an improvement in their symptoms within days of beginning treatment with dexamethasone; however, high doses of dexamethasone cannot be continued indefinitely because of the side effects that tend to become more pronounced with a longer duration of therapy.

Because dexamethasone suppresses normal hormone production by the adrenal gland, serious side effects can occur if you suddenly stop taking it. Follow your doctor's instructions exactly when taking dexamethasone or when tapering off it.

The side effects of dexamethasone vary with the dose and duration of use and also from patient to patient. Some of the most common side effects include weight gain, heartburn, fluid retention, muscle weakness, increased appetite, osteoporosis, insomnia, depression, nervousness, mania/mood swings, high blood sugar, low potassium, high blood pressure, thinning hair, rash

Corticosteroid

A naturally occurring hormone produced by the adrenal cortex, or a synthetic hormone having similar properties; often used to treat edema (swelling) in leaky capillaries of the brain.

or acne, thin skin, increased risk of infection, and cataracts.

Rapid withdrawal of dexamethasone may cause muscle and joint aches, low blood pressure, a loss of appetite, nausea and vomiting, low-grade fever, and headache. Sometimes it is necessary to continue the dose of dexamethasone at a constant level for a longer period to allow for recovery from steroid withdrawal symptoms. After recovery, your doctor will try to taper the drug at a slower rate.

Dexamethasone also can interact with many drugs, including anticonvulsants such as phenytoin (Dilantin) and phenobarbital. Dexamethasone may cause stomach upset when given with aspirin or nonsteroidal anti-inflammatory drugs such as ibuprofen (Advil).

M.L.'s comment:

When I was taking Decadron, the primary side effect that I experienced was weight gain. Just about everyone I know that has taken Decadron (or any steroid) has also experienced weight gain. Most people don't like to gain weight (myself included). To go through this experience is very frustrating; however, I had to just "suck it up" and realize that this was part of being sick. Frankly, I was happy to be alive, but the weight gain still bothered me at times. I think it's okay to be frustrated when the weight gain occurs, just as long as you don't let the frustration consume you. I have seen other patients' attitudes become so negative because of their weight gain. This isn't healthy. Just remember, the weight WILL COME OFF! I promise! I gained about 20 pounds or more, and eventually it all came off. I really had to work at losing the last 5 pounds, but I did lose it.

72. What are the side effects of anticonvulsant medication?

There are common, expected side effects of anticonvulsant medication and rare, life-threatening side effects. Follow your doctor's instructions exactly when taking anticonvulsants. Many of these drugs must be closely monitored with blood tests. **Table 6** lists anticonvulsants and their common and rare but serious side effects.

M.L.'s comment:

The side effects of anticonvulsant medication can vary depending on the kind that you're taking. For example, I took Dilantin for about 15 months, and the primary side effect that I experienced was fatigue. It's my understanding that this is a fairly common side effect to expect, and the extent of the fatigue will vary by individual. My neurologist was able to prescribe another medication called Provigil to assist with the fatigue that I experienced while on Dilantin. My husband called it my "picker upper" because that is exactly what it did. It really was wonderful in giving my body that boost of energy, and it kept me from feeling so tired at the end of the day.

After several months, I changed from Dilantin to a different medication called Keppra. Keppra doesn't cause the same level of fatigue that I was feeling with the Dilantin. In fact, I was able to stop using the Provigil that I was taking on a daily basis with the Dilantin.

My recommendation is that you talk to your neurologist regularly about how your anticonvulsant medications are making you feel because the side effects can vary with each person. Other medications can be prescribed in an effort to assist with your particular needs.

Here's a few tips that help me boost my energy when I'm feeling tired:

Table 6   Side Effects of Anticonvulsant Medication

	Common Side Effects	Rare but Serious Side Effects
Depakote (Valproic acid)	Drowsiness, nausea, tremor, and weight gain	Pancreatitis, hepatitis, and rash
Dilantin (Phenytoin)	Drowsiness, skin rash, dizziness, thickening of gums, nausea, constipation, and abnormal hair growth	Hepatitis, low blood counts, severe skin reaction, and fever enlarged lymph nodes
Felbatol (Felbamate)	Drowsiness, dizziness, nausea, tremors, trouble sleeping, and changes in taste	Rash or hives, jaundice, changes in vision, bleeding or bruising
Gabitril (Tiagabine)	Drowsiness, dizziness, fatigue, nervousness, diarrhea, indigestion, and mood swings	Lethargy, poor responsiveness, sore throat, and skin changes
Keppra (Levetiracetam)	Drowsiness, fatigue, dizziness, and loss of appetite	Flu-like symptoms and jaundice
Lamictal (Lamotrigine)	Drowsiness, skin rash, fatigue, nausea, difficulty sleeping, tremors, diarrhea or constipation	In children, severe skin rash which may be life-threatening; muscle pain, mouth sores, fever, swollen lymph nodes, and jaundice
Lyrica (Pregabalin)	Drowsiness, dizziness, fatigue, insomnia, weight gain, dry mouth, and constipation	Muscle jerks, breathing difficulty, chest pain, memory loss, and anxiety
Neurontin (Gabapentin)	Drowsiness, dizziness, fatigue, weight gain, constipation, and dry mouth	Visual disturbances, nausea, rash, tremor, and slurred speech
Phenobarbitol (Phenobarbitol)	Drowsiness, impaired cognition, reduced libido, nausea, and irritability	Hyperactivity, behavior changes, depression, jaundice, and headache
Tegretol (Carbamazepine) (Tegretol)	Drowsiness, dizziness, double vision, low blood counts, headache, and clumsiness	Visual disturbances, depression, skin rash, loss of coordination, stomach pain, and irregular heartbeat
Topamax (Topiramate)	Drowsiness, fatigue, psychomotor slowing, weight loss, depression, nausea, and altered taste	Speech disorders, kidney stones, difficulty breathing, and hearing loss
Trileptal (Oxcarbazepine)	Drowsiness, dizziness, and rash	Double vision and loss of coordination
Vimpat (Lacosamide)	Double vision, headache, nausea, and dizziness	Rarely, suicidal thoughts
Zonegran (Zonisamide)	Drowsiness, dizziness, loss of appetite, nausea, and weight loss	Hallucinations, difficulty breathing, kidney stones, rash, and mouth sores

- *When possible, try to incorporate some activity into your schedule. Even a short walk around the block will help get your blood moving and will give your body more energy.*
- *Take frequent breaks whenever possible.*
- *Eat as nutritiously as possible, and don't be afraid to eat. Food gives your body the fuel it needs to keep going.*
- *If a task doesn't have to be done right away, either don't do it or have someone else do it for you.*
- *Give yourself permission to stop when you're feeling tired. Take a nap if you need one. Listen to your body, and realize that it is okay to allow yourself to take it slow.*

73. My pharmacist said that there may be a "drug interaction" between some of my medications. What does this mean?

Many drugs undergo chemical changes in the body after intravenous or oral administration. When different drugs are used at the same time, one drug may affect the normal action of the other. Some drugs are chemically processed in the liver, but another drug used simultaneously may affect the normal processing of the first drug. In the case of both chemotherapy drugs and anticonvulsant drugs, the amount of the drug needed to produce the desired effect without toxicity (the therapeutic level) is very important.

Anticonvulsant drug interactions are particularly critical because the patient may have seizures if the therapeutic level drops. Some drugs will raise the anticonvulsant drug level, possibly resulting in a toxic level. Also, the use of an anticonvulsant drug may render the other drug partially or completely ineffective. Your pharmacist is trained to examine the list of your medications and look for possible drug interactions with your anticonvulsant. **Tables 7** and **8** list drug interactions with anticonvulsant and chemotherapy drugs.

Medications Used in Brain Tumor Treatment

Table 7   Drug Interactions with Anticonvulsant Medications

Dilantin	May interact with alcohol, benzodiazepines (valium, Klonopin), Coumadin, Tegretol, estrogens, Prozac, Ritalin, Thorazine, trazodone, doxycycline, steroids, aspirin, Bactrim, Depakote, vitamin D Reduces effectiveness of oral contraceptives
Phenobarbitol	May interact with alcohol, Dilantin, antihistamines, antidepressants, Ultram, Darvocet, muscle relaxants, steroids, sleeping pills Reduces effectiveness of oral contraceptives
Tegretol (Carbatrol)	May interact with alcohol, Prozac, ketoconazole, erythromycin, Phenobarbitol, Dilantin, Darvacet, Cardizem, Claritin, Depakote, Cisplatin, Coumadin, thyroid hormones, antifungals, methadone, steroids, Ultram, lithium Reduces effectiveness of oral contraceptives Increases risk of sunburn
Trileptal	May interact with Phenobarbitol, Dilantin, Depakote, Cardizem, Calan, cyclophosphamide, Vincristine, oral contraceptives
Felbatol	May interact with Tegretol, Phenobarbitol, Dilantin, Depakote, oral contraceptives, alcohol Increases risk of sunburn
Depakote	May interact with aspirin, Tegretol, Dilantin, Phenobarbitol, Lamical, Topomax, Coumadin, valium
Lamictal	May interact with Depakote, Tegretol, Dilantin, Phenobarbitol, Topomax, Bactrim, methotrexate, oral contraceptives, alcohol
Keppra	Avoid alcohol; use with caution when taking tricyclic antidepressants, Levaquin, Cipro
Topomax	Interacts with Dilantin, Tegretol, Depakote, Lamictal, Phenobarbitol, Elavil, lithium, sleeping pills, hydrochlorothiazide, digoxin, muscle relaxers Can reduce effectiveness of oral contraceptives
Neurontin, lyrica	Use with caution with alcohol, sedatives, morphine, antacids, naprosyn (Aleve), hydrocodone; oral diabetic medications (pioglitazone, rosglitazone)
Gabatril	May interact with Tegretol, Phenobarbitol, Dilantin, Depakote
Vimpat (Lacosamide)	Dilantin, Tegretol, and Phenobarbitol slightly reduce Vimpat levels
Zonegran	May interact with Phenobarbitol, Tegretol, and Dilantin; avoid alcohol

197

Table 8   Interactions of Chemotherapy with Other Treatments

BCNU (Carmustine) and CCNU (lomustine)	Radiation therapy Bone marrow depressants (chemotherapy, AZT, amphotericin B) Live virus vaccine Killed virus vaccine
Procarbazine (Matulane)	Alcohol, cocaine, antihistamines, anticonvulsants, antipsychotics, stimulants, levodopa, oral hypoglycemic drugs, caffeine, Prozac, Elavil, Buspar, Demerol, other narcotics, live virus vaccine, killed virus vaccine, green tea, Dilantin, trazodone, Ultram, dextromethorphan, cold medicines, antianxiety drugs, MAOI antidepressants
Temodar (Temozolomide)	Depakote, BCNU, CCNU, live virus vaccine
Etoposide (VP–16)	Cyclosporin, radiation therapy Live virus vaccine, killed virus vaccine
CPT–11 (Camptosar, irinotecan)	Radiation therapy, dexamethasone, diuretics (Lasix, Dyazide) oral hypoglycemic agents, chemotherapy (many), laxatives
Carboplatin (Paraplatin)	Dilantin, Phenobarbitol, Tegretol, Live virus vaccine, Killed virus Radiation therapy Aminoglycoside antibiotics (gentamicin, amikacin, tobramycin), live virus vaccine Killed virus vaccine
Cisplatin (Platinol)	Radiation therapy, aminoglycoside antibiotics, Tegretol, Depakote, Dilantin, Topamax, Phenobarbitol, Lamictal, Gabatril, Antivert, Compazine, Thorazine, antihistamines, bleomycin, live virus vaccine, killed virus vaccine
Methotrexate	Alcohol, Coumadin, non-steroidal anti-inflammatory drugs (NSAIDs); Aspirin, radiation therapy, Dilantin, Penicillins, Accutane, oral hypoglycemic agents, Bactrim, live virus vaccine, killed virus vaccine

It is also important that you continue the same anticonvulsant that your doctor prescribed; if you were told that you may only take the brand-name drug, for example, this is very important. Do not allow your insurance company to change your medication to a generic one without checking with your doctor first to see if this is allowed. This is more critical than with most other medications, as some generic medications are *not* equivalent to the brand-name medication. Also, be sure to note whether you are taking an "extended-release" formulation because switching to a drug with a shorter duration of effect could increase your risk of seizures. Chemotherapy can also interact with other medications.

74. I've never been depressed before, but since my diagnosis, I feel hopeless at times. Will an antidepressant help? Are there side effects that I need to consider if I'm on chemotherapy?

Depression in brain tumor patients can be related to the stress of the diagnosis and treatment, the loss of physical or mental capabilities, and the fear of suffering and death. For patients who have always enjoyed good health, the diagnosis of a brain tumor can be emotionally overwhelming. Almost all patients who are faced with serious illness experience at least temporary grief and anxiety about their condition, but some patients become so distraught that they are unable to make decisions regarding their own care. These patients may benefit from counseling or supportive psychotherapy with a medical professional who is experienced in helping patients with severe illness.

Severely depressed patients and patients with milder forms of depression may benefit from an antidepressant medication. Some of the newer antidepressant drugs,

Depression in brain tumor patients can be related to the stress of the diagnosis and treatment, the loss of physical or mental capabilities, and the fear of suffering and death.

known as selective serotonin reuptake inhibitors (SSRIs), include fluoxetine (Prozac), sertraline (Zoloft), paroxetine (Paxil), citalopram (Celexa), and escitalopram (Lexapro). These drugs have fewer side effects than the older tricyclic antidepressants such as amitriptyline (Elavil) and nortriptyline (Pamelor). Moreover, tricyclic antidepressants may increase the risk of seizures in some patients. Another antidepressant, bupropion (Wellbutrin; also known as Zyban when prescribed for smoking cessation), also increases the risk of seizures.

Patients who are taking procarbazine chemotherapy (one of the components of the popular combination PCV) need to be aware of potential drug interactions with antidepressant medications. Neither the SSRI drugs nor tricyclic antidepressants should be used by patients taking procarbazine.

Some patients resist the idea of taking antidepressant medication because of the large number of other medications they must take; however, studies have shown that cancer patients have an improvement in their overall quality of life when treated for depression. Studies also show that patients treated with antidepressants experience an increase in the number of natural killer cells, the cells that have an important role in the immune system.

75. Can I drink alcohol while taking chemotherapy or antiseizure medication?

Some drugs used in brain tumor therapy have known toxic reactions with alcohol; these include procarbazine, methotrexate, and thalidomide. Alcohol can interact with many other medications, including anticonvulsants (noted above), antidepressants, tranquilizers, sleeping pills, and pain medications. Activities that require concentration or coordination, such as driving, even after very small amounts of alcohol, should be strictly forbidden. Also, because of the increase in the sedating effect and duration of these drugs when combined with alcohol, accidental overdose and death are possible.

Patients taking anticonvulsants who also drink may experience wide fluctuations in drug levels, creating a risk of seizures or toxicity. Patients who drink alcohol with dinner each night, or as a "nightcap" who intend to continue this practice, must not assume that their physicians will approve of this practice. Also, it is common for patients to mislead their health care providers intentionally regarding their alcohol consumption or a history of alcoholism. It is extremely important that such information is presented honestly and, as with all health care information, is kept strictly confidential.

Although many patients can drink a glass of champagne at a wedding or sip a piña colada on the beach without risk, it is always recommended to inquire specifically whether any alcohol is allowed while taking chemotherapy or anticonvulsant drugs.

M.L.'s comment:

Personally, I would recommend that you NOT drink alcohol while taking chemotherapy. First, depending on the type of chemotherapy that you're taking, you'll probably experience fatigue as a side effect. Coupling alcohol with chemotherapy will make you even more tired. If you're like most people, you may experience fatigue with your antiseizure medication, and mixing alcohol with it will make you feel that much worse.

PART TEN

Living with a Brain Tumor

I have just learned that I have a brain tumor and I'm afraid. Is this common?

What dietary adjustments do I need to make during treatment? Should I take vitamin or mineral supplements? Can diet protect against the recurrence of a brain tumor?

Fatigue is a big problem for me. I simply don't have the energy to do anything. What can I do about this?

More . . .

76. I have just learned that I have a brain tumor and I'm afraid. Is this common?

Yes. Most people who are diagnosed with serious illness grapple with fear and anxiety. Some patients fear physical disability, loss of income, loss of health insurance, or loss of support from their family. Some patients fear surgery, radiation therapy, or other treatment. Some patients fear that they will die. The majority of people fear what they cannot control, and there are many aspects of brain tumors that are unpredictable and uncontrollable.

Not all brain tumors are life threatening. Some can be cured surgically, and some can be controlled for long periods of time with radiation therapy or chemotherapy. Learning about your condition may help you to cope with your fear. If you fear specific aspects of your treatment, tell your doctor so that you can receive help in coping with your treatment.

M.L.'s comment:

If you aren't afraid, then you aren't normal! I was feeling great; I was about to get promoted to vice president. My husband and I were talking about starting a family. I didn't have any warning signs at all. Then I woke up one morning, and I didn't feel well. The next thing I knew, I was told that I had a brain tumor. Frankly, I didn't know what that really meant. My husband did a great deal of research on the Internet to find out as much as he could about brain tumors. I was scared, but there seemed to be this voice inside of me that kept telling me that I would be okay. I had read at one time that "cancer is NOT a death sentence," and I believed that.

Having faith in God and believing I would be taken care of also helped to ease my fears. Someone told me once that faith was the most effective antidote for fear. That proved to be true in my situation. Others have suggested that hope is the most effective antidote for fear. I'm sure there are many different opinions about what is considered effective for fighting the battle with cancer. I just continued to believe that I would be okay and that I would make it through all of this.

My husband, friends, and family were all an incredible support system for me. Believe me—I was depressed at times, too. There were times when I cried a lot. About 3 or 4 months after my surgery—when I was well into my radiation treatments—I seemed to be very emotional for a period of several weeks. When my mother or my sister would call me to see how I was doing, I would just start to cry. I think the reality of the situation had set in. My doctors told me that the depression could have also been associated with my medication.

Based on everything that I have either felt myself, read elsewhere, or heard from others, it's perfectly natural to have negative feelings about the diagnosis that you've been given. You have to deal with the fact that your life has changed. You'll probably experience other feelings, such as denial and resentment. During the initial stages, you'll probably become somewhat numb to it all. Again, all of this is normal. I experienced all of these feelings; however, at some point after the reality of the situation set in, I realized how important it was for me to think about how I could take those negative feelings and turn them into positive energy. For some reason, I kept thinking that this happened to me for a reason. My husband kept thinking, "Why M.L.?" and "What has she done in her life to deserve this?"

Eventually, a sense of acceptance set in that changed the way we lived our lives from that moment on. Duane and I did talk openly about my diagnosis and how it changed our lives. I needed him to tell me many of the details that took place early on because I couldn't remember them. Duane was terrified that he was going to lose me within the first year of my diagnosis. I felt like I had to be strong for him because he was so worried that he would lose me. I think the thought of me not being the "same M.L." scared him almost as much as the thought of losing me completely. We talked about all of these feelings, and we allowed ourselves to be unhappy while we were having these discussions. We always tried to end such discussions on a positive note. We'd say that we would fight this one day at a time and deal with whatever was given to us.

This whole situation actually brought Duane and I closer. We were very close before, but coping with news of this magnitude was something that neither of us had ever had to do. We found that we clung to one another for support and strength. I also found a great deal of comfort and strength in my religion. The church and my pastor were there for me and prayed for me all the time. I can't even begin to tell you how many people told me they were praying for me, and I believe that a person who gets prayed for gets well more quickly.

Since my diagnosis, I feel like my personal life has changed for the better. I've heard others say the same thing. I think it's because you're forced to take a good look at how your life was before the diagnosis of a brain tumor. You're given a chance to re-evaluate your life and make changes for the better. I started trying to figure out what "message was being sent to me" and what I was supposed to do with the message I received. I sometimes wonder if this all happened because it was a way to get me to help other people with brain tumors. By sharing my story of dealing with a malignant brain tumor, I could help others be more positive about their situations. I've thought about this so many times, and every time I get a different answer. These days, I just try to do the best I can to live a good life. I try to be a good influence on others who may be coping with some of the same issues that I experienced with a brain tumor.

77. What dietary adjustments do I need to make during treatment? Should I take vitamin or mineral supplements? Can diet protect against the recurrence of a brain tumor?

Dietary adjustments may be necessary, but recommendations vary from patient to patient. For example, patients who have nausea and vomiting may need to change their eating habits. Fried, spicy, or sweet foods may be more upsetting to your stomach when you feel nauseated. Cold foods tend to be better tolerated than hot foods.

Some patients develop mouth ulcers or yeast in the mouth or throat during treatment. The presence of yeast (candidiasis) can affect taste, contributing to loss of appetite. Report to your doctor any painful sores in the mouth and throat that limit eating and drinking. Specific medical treatment for the sores as well as nutritional beverages such as Ensure or Prosure can help to keep you from losing weight during treatment and may be recommended.

Although regular consumption of fruits and vegetables is recommended, patients with very low white blood cell counts may need to avoid raw or uncooked foods because they may still have bacteria in them.

Supplemental vitamins and minerals are not required in a well-balanced diet; however, many patients suffer

Dietary adjustments may be necessary, but recommendations vary from patient to patient.

nausea, poor appetite, or fatigue, which can affect their ability to cook and eat a balanced diet. Although multivitamins and iron supplements provide essential nutrients, patients under treatment must also consume enough calories and protein. Your doctor may refer you to a dietician if your nutritional needs are not being met and you are losing weight.

Unfortunately, keeping well-nourished and physically healthy does not guarantee that you will avoid a relapse. There are no known modifications of diet that will achieve or prolong remission in brain tumor patients; however, keeping healthy will allow better tolerance of subsequent treatment.

Many cancer patients have been told to avoid sugar in any form because of the concern that "sugar feeds cancer." Unfortunately, it is not that simple. Patients who have eliminated sugar completely from their diets do not find that this has "starved" their tumor. The consumption of refined sugar and other carbohydrates may crowd out more nutritious foods, and for this reason, patients are encouraged to keep sugars and carbohydrates to a minimum. Some patients have poor appetite, nausea, mouth sores, and other problems that limit their food intake. These patients may derive benefit from protein shakes, "smoothies," and other high-calorie drinks.

Your oncologist or oncology nurse can help you to modify your diet if you experience weight loss, weight gain, nausea, or diarrhea. Make sure that you discuss your diet with your physician before eliminating meat, vegetables, fruit, or other classes of nutrients. Many excellent books have been written for cancer patients, often with recipes for patients undergoing chemotherapy.

78. Fatigue is a big problem for me. I simply don't have the energy to do anything. What can I do about this?

Fatigue is a common problem for cancer patients. In fact, two-thirds of patients report fatigue severe enough to limit their daily activities. Fatigue is not the same as weakness (a loss of strength), but fatigue does involve a sense of generalized weakness, impaired concentration, and tiring easily. Fatigue can be associated with anemia (a low red blood cell count), neutropenia (a low neutrophil count), pain, depression, anxiety, and a loss of appetite. Treatment of these factors can sometimes improve the sense of fatigue.

Fatigue can be associated with cancer treatment such as radiation therapy and chemotherapy. The latter can cause anemia and neutropenia. The feeling of fatigue may lessen when the blood count returns to normal. In addition, correcting low blood counts with growth factors such as Procrit (for anemia) and Neupogen (for neutropenia) may allow chemotherapy to continue at the recommended doses.

Fatigue can be associated with cancer treatment such as radiation therapy and chemotherapy.

Cancer patients with normal blood counts may still complain of fatigue. **Table 9** lists other causes of fatigue. Make sure that you discuss the feeling of fatigue with your doctor. It is particularly important to note accompanying symptoms such as shortness of breath, constipation, nausea, and muscle weakness, which may have a separate, treatable cause.

Strategies for combating fatigue include the following:

- Participating in aerobic exercise and physical activity
- Keeping a normal sleep/wake cycle
- Planning a rest period following physical exertion

Table 9   Causes of Fatigue in Cancer Patients

Types of Fatigue	Possible Cause
Cancer-related	Post-operative/post-anesthesia Presence of cancer Radiation therapy Chemotherapy
Nutrition-related	Hypoglycemia (low blood pressure) Weight loss Weight gain secondary to steroids
Related to a mood disorder	Depression Anxiety
Related to another illness	Infection/Fever Heart disease Lung disease Thyroid disease Chronic pain
Medication-related	Anticonvulsants Pain medication Sedatives Rapid steroid taper

- Setting limits on strenuous work activities
- Conserving energy for specific activities
- Managing stress
- Avoiding foods with a high sugar content

Finally, certain vitamin and mineral deficiencies can contribute to fatigue. Supplemental vitamins may be recommended in these cases; however, supplemental vitamins for patients who do not have these deficiencies do not help and could even be harmful.

79. Now that my treatment is over, why am I not happy about it—or at least relieved?

M.L.'s comment:

First, you should keep in mind that your treatments may not end at some fixed point in time. I thought that because the visible tumor was removed during my craniotomy and because I had received radiation treatments successfully that my chemotherapy treatments would be "short-lived." After receiving treatments for 12 months, I was presented with a number of different options, one of which was to discontinue treatments. After looking at all of the information, my husband and I decided that it would be best for me to continue with my treatments.

Even though I continued with the treatments, I still had many questions such as, "What if my tumor starts to come back even though I stay on chemo?" or "How long will I have to be on chemotherapy?" and "What will the effects be on the rest of my body if I stay on chemotherapy?" These are tough questions to get answers to because ultimately the decisions must be made by you and your loved ones. The doctors can provide you with some of the answers, but they have to be careful not to tell you what to do. To this day, I still struggle with wanting to know the answer to, "Will I have to take certain medications forever?"

If you aren't happy or relieved when your treatment ends, remember that this is a very common and normal experience. Most people who battle brain cancer have a fear of recurrence. This fear is especially difficult to deal with when treatment ends because your health care team is no longer surrounding you on a regular basis. There is a natural sense of loss and fear, but you can't allow the fear to take control of your life. Remember that you are in control of your emotions. Part of that control is to be aware of your fears. Don't let your fears dictate the way you live your life.

You have probably realized that you can't control your future, but you can have a positive attitude and live one day at a time. This is a great time to get involved in brain tumor support groups if you haven't already. You can share your fears and emotions with other members of the support group, and there is a very good chance that those same fears and emotions have been felt by other members of the group.

You should also remember that your family and friends are still there for you, even after your treatment ends. Don't be afraid to share your feelings with them and to look to them for support and understanding. Also, make sure that you take the time to do the things that you enjoy. All you can do is live one day at a time, but don't be afraid to seek professional help for counseling if you feel that your fears have become excessive.

I mentioned this earlier in Part Three regarding MRI [magnetic resonance imaging] scans, but I will repeat it here, as it is one of the best pieces of advice that I received from a support group. One of the counselors said to me, "If you cannot change the outcome of a situation, then DO NOT worry about it." If you think about that statement, it makes a lot of sense, and it has really stuck with me over the years. I find myself practicing this in many areas of my life. One in particular is when it is time for my next MRI scan. For example, there isn't a thing I can do to change the outcome of my MRI scan, so I do not worry about the results. If the results come back and they are not 100% positive, then I know there will be options for me to discuss with my neuro-oncologist. You might think that sounds a bit too simplistic, but if you find yourself worrying about your future, then I would encourage you to first think about what you can and cannot control. If you cannot change the outcome, then do not worry about it because worrying about something that you cannot change will only cause more stress and fear. If you focus your efforts on situations or outcomes that you CAN change, then you will be directing your energy in a positive way and hopefully will find that your stress levels will decrease significantly.

80. I didn't need physical therapy after my surgery, but I've always been physically active. Can I resume regular exercise?

M.L.'s comment:

The answer to this question depends on your particular situation. I would recommend you consult your doctor; however, in my opinion, you should strive to begin or resume some sort of exercise as soon as your doctor approves. When I started exercising again, I felt that I needed to do it in order to assist in my rehabilitation. I felt like the exercise was helping me to keep up my strength. I remember my doctor telling me that it was good to exercise because it is dangerous to be too sedentary, even in the postoperative period. She told me that if patients don't stay active, they are at a higher risk for blood clots in their legs. I was also eager to start exercising because the steroids that I took contributed to my loss of muscle strength. I was happy to be able to start exercising so that I could gain back that strength.

Keep in mind that exercise can be anything from a walk around the block to spending 30 minutes on an exercise bike. When I started exercising again, I didn't try to overdo it. I just wanted to be able to resume some sort of activity. If my doctor told me I could start out with a walk around the block and no more, then that is what I did. As I was able to regain my strength, I was able to gradually increase my level of exercise.

Another bonus is that people who exercise generally feel better mentally as well as physically. I think this is particularly true when someone fears that they have lost strength or coordination after surgery. Working to regain strength and flexibility is an important part of getting well.

81. Will I be allowed to drive?

Driving is clearly a complex task that requires multitasking on a level that many adults take for granted. For parents who have had a teenager learning to drive, the anxiety of allowing a 16-year-old access to the family car is well understood. Will your teenager anticipate all of the hazards on the highway, the stopping distance, and the noise distractions within the car? Insurance companies, of course, know that learning to drive is difficult, which is why rates for young drivers are typically high.

Relearning to drive is no less difficult when a patient has undergone surgery for a brain tumor. Although there may not be apparent motor weakness, visual abnormalities, or blind spots, patients may have slower reaction times and a decreased ability to note subtle environmental clues in traffic. Many neurosurgeons do not allow patients to drive for 6 weeks after surgery. Some neurosurgeons recommend that patients permanently surrender their driver's licenses.

Patients who have suffered seizures, even without loss of consciousness, are restricted from driving.

Patients who have suffered seizures, even without loss of consciousness, are restricted from driving. In some states, the patient must be seizure-free for a least 1 year. The doctor must document that the patient has been counseled regarding driving. Doctors who do allow their brain tumor patients to drive often only recommend drives that are absolutely necessary and involve limited distance, light traffic, and good visibility.

There are rehabilitation programs that perform an assessment of driving using either a simulator or an actual road test under controlled conditions. Reaction time, attention to traffic, judgment of stopping distance, and depth perception are all important facets of relearning to drive.

82. How should I tell my family, friends, and young children about my diagnosis?

M.L.'s comment:

Telling someone that you have a brain tumor isn't an easy thing to do. In many cases, however, it can be more helpful for you to share your situation with those who care about you the most. They can be there to provide support and also help you to make some of the tough decisions that you'll face. Because there are so many different brain tumor types, I found it necessary to share a great deal of information with my family and friends so that they really understood how serious my illness was. My husband was incredible when it came to this aspect of talking about my situation. He helped me find out as much as possible about brain tumors by gathering information from the doctors as well as the Internet.

My husband told my parents about my brain tumor, and then my parents informed the rest of my family. Fortunately, my parents have medical backgrounds, and thus, they could relay the information accurately. If necessary, your doctors and other medical support staff can offer support when you tell your family and friends about your illness. In my case, my parents continued to provide updates to the rest of my family because they all live in Tennessee.

I remember my husband telling me about how he told some of our closest friends, Gil and Jayne. Gil's a real tough guy on the outside, but he was very upset. Jayne was really depressed and couldn't talk about it without starting to cry, but both of them were there for us no matter how hard it was for them. Gil was great because he always tries to be positive. When appropriate, he would try to interject a little humor somewhere just to keep us laughing. I'll never forget when he came to the hospital wearing black jeans and a black shirt. Duane later told me that Gil had taken a piece of paper and stuck it in his collar so that he appeared to be a priest. It was hard not to laugh at him pretending to be a priest! As soon Gil took the fake Roman collar out, my real pastor arrived at the hospital to see me. It is a good thing that my pastor has a great sense of humor.

In many cases, when I told a friend that I had a brain tumor I found it easiest to get straight to the point and just say, "I was recently diagnosed with a brain tumor." After they got over the shock of what I said, I found the support from them to be overwhelming.

I will also say that although so many people were supportive, there were a few friends who seemed almost uncomfortable in dealing with my illness and being there for me. At first this hurt my feelings, but I later learned that this is a common occurrence. There wasn't a thing I could do to change it. I just came to the realization that many people just don't know what to say, or perhaps dealing with my illness may have reminded them of a sad situation that they may have previously experienced. I decided not to let it get to me and focused on the fact that I had many more friends who were able to be there with me. That is what was important.

With regard to telling your children that you have a brain tumor, I should begin by letting you know that I don't have children of my own; however, I do have a good friend with a brain tumor, and she does have children. I have talked to her quite a bit about this subject and have also seen and read information that is intended to be helpful when telling young children that you have a brain tumor. The following comments summarize what I have been told by my friend or have found to be consistent with information that I have found in other sources.

First, always be honest with your children. If your children sense that something unusual is happening, then they may use their imagination to create a problem if they aren't told the truth. If that happens, what their minds may invent may be much worse than the truth. You'll need to address the children's concerns and talk with them in words that they understand. I have been told that if a brain tumor is described fairly simply to young children (e.g., "Daddy has a lump in his head that isn't supposed to be there"), then it is easier for them to understand. They need to understand what it means for you to go to the hospital or perhaps have to stay in the hospital for a while. Most people that I have spoken to have suggested that a parent needs to answer a child's questions honestly and simply in words that are most appropriate for the child's age. Talking with your children in a loving, truthful, and reassuring manner is essential to their sense of security.

Second, be aware of your timing; it's best to talk to your children as soon after your diagnosis as possible. Tell your children as much as you think they need to know in order to calm their fears, but not necessarily everything. In other words, too much information may cause them to worry about things that they can't change. The older the child, the more information you should provide.

Tell your children that you may have treatments that may cause you to lose your hair and make you feel tired. It's okay to tell them that these things are not normal but are part of the process of dealing with a brain tumor. If you're going to have surgery to remove the tumor, you should share this information with them as well. Again, what you say and how you say it will depend on the age of the children. Your children also need to know that having a brain tumor and the signs and symptoms that go with it isn't their fault. Let them know that they can't "catch" your condition by being close to you or touching you.

Don't forget to ask your children if they have any questions. You may be surprised by their concerns, but keep in mind that you also need to be prepared to answer their questions. They may ask you if you're going to die. Your response will depend on the age and maturity of your children. Your specific condition will also be a factor in your response. Once again, you must be truthful with them, but you must always encourage them to be hopeful. Help your children understand that a person who has a brain tumor doesn't necessarily die from it.

A friend of mine told me that she felt that it was important to tell her children's teachers. The teachers and school counselors were very supportive and helped her to better understand how her children were coping with the situation.

Finally, it's okay if you start to cry when you are telling your children. Crying is a very normal reaction when talking to your children about your situation. Just make sure that you tell them why you're crying. It may be because you're sad that you're sick or that you are nervous about some of the changes that may take place as a result of your illness. You should always reassure your children that you'll talk to them about what is happening to you and that you will do everything you can to make sure that their needs are taken care of by family and friends. Remember to encourage your children to stay positive and to be hopeful.

One change in communication that has evolved since the first edition of this book is the use of web logs, or blogs, to keep everyone informed about the patient's course. Now that friends and family are often spread out across the country or even around the world, keeping everyone up to date with short posts can be very helpful. One patient I knew literally had hundreds of coworkers and colleagues and former colleagues who were all very interested in his progress and eager to support him through it. He was even able to learn of new treatment options as people forwarded articles they had read about current research. Another patient, Jerry Kline, has used his website (www.jerrykline.com) not only to keep his friends and family up to date, but to reach out to other brain tumor patients to encourage them.

83. My caregiver is experiencing feelings of anger, frustration, sadness, and guilt. Where can caregivers go to get help?

M.L.'s comment:

While most will say "the patient comes first," and that is a true statement, let us not forget about the caregiver. In fact, Dr. Paul Zeltzer has been noted as saying, "Caregivers are the most important member of the health care team"; however, many times the caregiver tends to be forgotten. More often than not the caregiver is the one that is juggling everything from the emotional support and personal care to appointments and insurance issues.

Typically, a caregiver is a family member, perhaps a spouse, sibling, parent, or a close friend. Over time, there can be multiple caregivers; however, most of the time there is one primary caregiver.

As a brain tumor patient AND a caregiver (for my father), I have to say that the challenges and frustration that I experienced as a caregiver were much more difficult than those as a patient. Some of the best "caregiver" advice that I read was that it is important for caregivers to not lose sight of ways to take care of themselves, in addition to the person/patient that you are caring for.

It occurred to me that it is not difficult, and in many situations is recommended, to obtain a second opinion or find another doctor, but it's not so easy to get another caregiver!

The American Brain Tumor Association (ABTA) has an entire section on their website that is dedicated to support, advice, and additional resources for caregivers (www.abta.org/ Care_And_Support/48). In addition, there is a section that has extensive detail with regard to orientation for caregivers and a free handbook for family caregivers of patients with brain tumors. Go to the ABTA site to download individual chapters or the entire document.

As a caregiver for my father, some of the information and articles that I found especially useful at the ABTA website were as follows:

- *Advice to the Caregiver: Provides excellent advice and guiding principles to live by such as:*
  - *Shock: Allowing yourself to be in it and how to find a way out of it.*
  - *Crying: It is okay to cry, and crying is encouraged.*
  - *Hope and Prayer: Both of these provide strength and courage.*
- *Care for the Caregiver: The focus is on how caregivers can care for themselves using suggestions such as these:*
  - *Laughter: How this can ease tension and promote relaxation.*
  - *Be kind and patient to yourself.*
  - *Take care of yourself: Physical, health and emotional needs.*
- *Orientation to Caregiving Handbook: This is for family caregivers of patients with brain tumors. This resource helps caregivers understand brain tumors, what to expect, how to care for a loved one, paying for health care, planning for the future, and much more. This is an excellent resource to read or download or have sent by mail, if preferred.*

- *ABTA's Pen Pal Program: This program helps to connect brain tumor patients or caregivers with others who are in a similar situation.*

84. I'm concerned about the cost of my treatment since I lost my insurance. What can I do?

M.L.'s comment:

Clearly, the financial burden that is associated with having cancer will be somewhat less painful if you have insurance; however, options are available for those who do not have insurance. You should speak with the hospital or clinic, as it will be able to provide contacts regarding financial case workers or social workers who have more information about places to go for help. Also, other organizations may be available to provide assistance such as government programs, disability benefits, or volunteer organizations.

I would strongly recommend that you check the American Brain Tumor Association website (www.abta.org), as it has a list of extremely useful resources and websites in the "Care and Support" section. I have listed some information here; however, there is so much information on the ABTA website as it is not possible to list it all here.

I would suggest you start here with the following:

Financial Assistance Resources and Websites

Medical Care

- *Supplemental Security Income (SSI) and Social Security Disability Insurance (SSDI), 800-772-1213, www.socialsecurity.gov. Contact your local Social Security Office to determine whether you qualify for SSI or SSDI. The medical requirements and disability determination process* are the same under both programs. Eligibility for SSDI is based on prior work under Social Security, whereas SSI is based on financial need.

- *Hill-Burton Funds, 800-638-0742, www.hrsa.gov/hill-burton/hillburtonfacilities.htm.* Hill-Burton Funds are federal grants that allow hospitals and nursing homes to provide low- or no-cost medical care to those meeting income guidelines. Contact Hill-Burton to receive a listing of hospitals or nursing homes participating in the program. Funding and sites are limited.

- *U.S. Department of Health and Human Services Bureau of Primary Health Care, 888-275-4772, http://bphc. hrsa.gov.* This agency provides information on public programs for the uninsured.

Prescription Drugs

- *Patient Advocate Foundation, 866-512-3861, www. copays.org.* Their Co-Pay Relief Program offers copayment assistance to patients with brain cancer. The program accepts calls beginning the first of each month until funds are depleted. The providers can also apply on behalf of their patients online.

- *Partnership for Prescription Assistance, 888-477-2669, www.pparx.org.* This organization offers a single point of access to more than 475 public, state, and private patient assistance programs, including more than 180 programs offered by pharmaceutical companies.

Utilities

- *Low-Income Home Energy Assistance Program, 866 674-6327, www.acf.hhs.gov/programs/ocs/liheap/index.html.* This program helps low-income households meet their home energy needs.

Gasoline Assistance

- *Free Gas USA, Inc., www.freegasusa.org.* A nationwide nonprofit assistance program for low-income people *having trouble paying for gasoline. Applications can be made for gas grant cards that range in value from $50 to $1,200, depending on need and circumstances. In order to be eligible for a gas card, a person's yearly income must be at or below the "very low limit" category as defined by the U.S. Department of HUD. An income calculator is available at the website. Applications are available and must be substantiated by a human service agency, and applicants must be a resident of the United States.*

Medical Supplies

- *The Cancer Fund of America, 800-578-5284, www.cfoa. org. Provides for nonprescription medical needs such as nutritional supplements or incontinence supplies. Items available vary as the group receives donated products from companies. Patients or family members can call and be placed in their database for specific needs.*

General Financial Assistance

- *Mission4Maureen, www.mission4maureen.com. Mission4 Maureen is dedicated to providing financial assistance to families who are burdened with the staggering cost of brain cancer treatment. Financial aid is available for medical bills as well as child care, housing payments, utility bills, transportation, medication, and other areas of assistance. An application with supporting documentation is required.*
- *National Brain Tumor Society, 800-934-2873, www. braintumor.org. This organization typically provides grants between $100 to $500 to financially needy brain tumor patients to help with treatment and symptom-related expenses, including transportation. Also included are costs associated with child care, home adaptations, and home health assistance.*
- *Netwish, www.netwish.org, provides assistance up to $500 for those who are able to demonstrate a financial need.*

Food Programs

- *Angel Food Ministries is a nonprofit, nondenominational organization dedicated to providing grocery relief and financial support to communities throughout the United States. Participants can purchase groceries at a reduced cost through one of their host sites. There are currently sites in 32 different states. Visit their website at: www.angelfoodministries.com or call 877-366-3646 to see whether there is a program near you.*

Programs for Children

- *Cancer Recovery Program, 800-238-6479, www. CancerRecovery.org. The Children's Project provides gift bags, camp scholarships, and limited emergency funding to pediatric oncology patients under the age of 18 years in the United States.*
- *Friends4Michael Foundation, 845-774-4809, www. friends4michael.org. This foundation provides nonmedical financial assistance to brain tumor patients up to the age of 18 years at the time of diagnosis, and who are currently undergoing medical treatment. Requests must be submitted by a social worker.*
- *St. Jude Children's Research Hospital, 901-495-3300, www.stjude.org. St. Jude offers treatment protocols for pediatric brain tumors. All patients accepted are treated without regard to the family's ability to pay. Referral must be made through a physician.*
- *United Healthcare Children's Foundation, 952-992-4459, www.unitedhealthcarechildrensfoundation.org. UHCF offers financial assistance to cover medical services beyond what insurance will cover or if service is not covered by the policy at all. Children who are U.S. citizens and are currently covered under a commercial health insurance policy are eligible up to the age of 17 years. Generally, assistance must be requested before services are obtained, and funds will*

generally be paid directly to the facility. UHCF grants up to $5,000 per year, with a lifetime cap of $7,500.

Miscellaneous Programs

- *Cleaning for a Reason, 877-337-3348, www.cleaning-forareason.org. This nonprofit organization offers free professional housecleaning services to improve the lives of women undergoing treatment for cancer. It provides once-a-month cleaning for 4 months. It is currently available in approximately 40 states and Canada.*
- *National Foundation of Dentistry for the Handicapped, 303-534-5360, www.nfdh.org. This organization offers a Donated Dental Services (DDS) program. DDS tends to the dental needs of the disabled, elderly, or medically compromised individuals who cannot afford the necessary dental treatment. Their website offers contact information for each state to help you locate a participating program in your area.*

General Information

- *Patient Advocate Foundation, 800-532-5274, www.PatientAdvocate.org. The website offers a state-by-state directory of information for patients seeking financial relief for a broad range of needs, including housing, utilities, food, transportation to medical treatment, and children's resources. Click on Resources, then Publications, and finally, The National Financial Resources Guidebook for Patients, to search this directory.*
- *The American Cancer Society also has helpful information on their website (www.cancer.org) regarding Medicaid and Medicare eligibility.*

85. Is it possible to get pregnant while on chemotherapy?

Yes, it is possible; however, it is very important to avoid pregnancy during chemotherapy and radiation therapy.

Exposure to radiation therapy and chemotherapy, particularly early in pregnancy, is associated with a high risk to the fetus.

Exposure to radiation therapy and chemotherapy, particularly early in pregnancy, is associated with a high risk to the fetus. Even later in pregnancy, chemotherapy may cause low birth weight and low blood counts in the unborn child.

Reliable contraception is recommended for all women of childbearing potential while undergoing treatment for a brain tumor. Chemotherapy can induce temporary or permanent infertility, and many female patients experience a change in their menstrual cycles while receiving chemotherapy. Some patients experience premature menopause (their periods never return), and some resume their periods and normal fertility after chemotherapy.

A waiting period of several months after treatment with chemotherapy is also recommended for women who are considering pregnancy. This allows for recovery from the side effects of therapy. For women whose menstrual periods return to normal and are able to conceive, there does not appear to be an increased risk of birth defects.

86. If I return to work at my desk job while I'm on chemotherapy, will I have to take any special precautions?

Returning to work is a positive experience for many people who may have been away for several weeks after surgery or other treatment; however, most patients find that they are more fatigued than expected and may require more frequent breaks or a shorter work schedule. Even with a desk job, it is common to feel exhausted at the end of the day.

In addition to adequate rest, getting regular exercise and good nutrition are important for maintaining a sense of well-being while on chemotherapy. Patients who have nausea from their chemotherapy may be able to arrange their work schedules to allow more time off after chemotherapy. They may also be able to take nonsedating antiemetic medication.

Some patients on chemotherapy have low blood counts and are at risk for infection. Working closely with co-workers who may be ill or in rooms with poor ventilation may increase the risk of infection. Antibacterial soaps or hand wipes may help limit the transmission of infection in the workplace.

87. Friends, coworkers, and neighbors who have heard about my brain tumor offer to help, but I'm not sure what I should tell them. What do caregivers and loved ones need to know in order to best support a person with a brain tumor?

M.L.'s comment:

First, patients and caregivers need to know that they shouldn't be afraid to ask for help! It's highly likely that you have many family and friends who want to help. Now is the time to let them. Even though my family lived out of town, it seemed as though there wasn't a day that went by that I didn't talk to my mother or father or someone else in my family. Having to be separated by hundreds of miles was hard on all of us, but being able to at least talk on the phone helped me get through some of my toughest days. Some of our friends provided not only moral support, but also practical help when we needed it the most. For example, when my parents came in town to be with me for several weeks for my surgery and recovery, one of my closest friends took my mother to the salon so that she could get her hair done. The help that we received from our friends gave my husband more time to be with me. They also helped to relieve some of the stress that comes along with feeling that the caregiver must be responsible for everything.

Our friends continued to be there for not only me, but also for my husband, Duane. There were times when I don't know what he would have done without having his best buddy there to just listen, be sympathetic, and give him as much support as he could on how to deal with some of his fears and concerns about me. I also felt very fortunate to have the support of colleagues and senior executives at work.

One of the greatest things that the president of the division I was working in said to me was that I didn't need to worry about anything regarding my work responsibilities and taking time off. He told me that I had given more than 15 years of my life to the company, and now it was time for the company to give some of that time back to me. It's difficult to express the peace of mind those words gave to me. Receiving such support from one of the most senior executives at my company allowed Duane and me to focus completely on the treatments that would help me get better.

As I started to get better, we would have our friends over. Just being able to share good news and bad news with family members or close friends provided so much support. Duane and I could tell that it was important to them to understand what we were going through. Our family and friends were there to listen, offer advice, and sometimes assist us in getting additional information.

88. I was diagnosed with a brain tumor over 5 years ago, and I still have problems with fatigue, short-term memory, and occasional seizures. How can I make my family and friends understand these problems? They seem to think that because the tumor hasn't come back I should be able to do everything that I used to.

First, it is important to explain to them (or have your doctor explain to them) that a long-term remission is a wonderful blessing, but it is not a "return to normal." In addition to damage caused by the tumor, surgery and treatment can also cause long-term effects. Some effects, as you point out, may not get better over time. This is something that has to be accepted. As with many other chronic conditions, you cannot "will" yourself back to your previous physical condition, memory, or level of energy.

It may be that your family members want to deny your symptoms because they think that acknowledging your limitations will make you dwell on the tumor and become depressed. They may be aware of your limitations but do not want to seem to pity you. Regardless of the reasons, remember that you cannot control what others think or do. You can only deal with your situation as well as you can.

It may help to ask your doctor for a referral to a family counselor. Also, if you have a trusted friend who can discuss your feelings with your family as your advocate, you may ask him or her to intervene on your behalf. Finally, you should consider discussing your feelings with other brain tumor patients, as you can draw

If you have a trusted friend who can discuss your feelings with your family as your advocate, you may ask him or her to intervene on your behalf.

Living with a Brain Tumor

strength and support from others who have experienced similar situations.

M.L.'s comment:

Another situation could occur and that is that YOU think you can do everything you used to be able to do. As a 9-year brain cancer survivor, that is something that I struggle with all of the time. It could be that I don't get enough sleep or I don't eat right. There are also many times when I forget to take a break during the day after I've spent several hours in front of my computer working on a project. I think the most frustrating thing for me is when I cannot "find the word" that I want to use when speaking with someone. I know that is a side effect of having a brain tumor. At such times, I try to remind myself that I had a life-threatening disease, and I'm doing well now, far better than I thought I would be able to do. This helps me take the small frustrations in stride and be grateful for what I do have.

PART ELEVEN

Taking Control of Your Future

Are there specific support groups for brain tumor patients? How do I find one?

What records do I need to keep about my treatment? What is the best way to stay organized?

My oncologist told me that even though I'm doing well, my tumor will probably come back at some point. He said, "Hope for the best, but prepare for the worst." I'm hoping for the best, but how do I prepare for the worst?

More . . .

89. Are there specific support groups for brain tumor patients? How do I find one?

M.L.'s comment:

Yes, many good support groups are available for brain tumor patients. Some people think that all support groups are the same, but that isn't necessarily true. I have been to a number of different support groups and have found that each of them are as different as the people who are in them. Brain tumor support groups can provide an opportunity to share practical information, offer wisdom, or hear other stories of survival. I would strongly recommend that if you're interested in attending a brain tumor support group, you should do so. Support groups can provide tremendous benefit for the patient and the caregiver. Plan to try out a group a few times. If you don't like a particular group, try another one.

To locate a support group in your area, contact the American Brain Tumor Association (www.abta.org) or the American Cancer Society (www.cancer.org). Both of these are excellent places to start.

There are too many resources to list here; however, you can

- *Ask your doctor, nurse, or social worker*
- *Ask your cancer treatment center or hospital*
- *Check your local newspaper or telephone book*
- *Ask others that you may know with brain cancer*

Other support groups are excellent and are not directed at a specific type of cancer or even a specific disease. Gilda's Club, for example, is a national organization with a number of locations across the United States. Gilda's Club, named in honor of Gilda Radner, sponsors special events, classes, exercise programs, and other activities. The Wellness Community, an organization that also has nationwide chapters, is another helpful resource for patients and families.

If you live in an area that doesn't have a support group for cancer patients, it's still possible to get information and support from brain tumor chat rooms on the Internet. This can be a bit tricky, as some people have a tendency to offer medical advice based on their own experience, but it can still be a positive experience for patients and caregivers.

It's also possible, of course, to start your own support group. If you know other patients in your community, let them know that you're interested in starting an informal discussion group. You may want to host a meeting in your home or ask a hospital or a church to let you use a meeting room once a month. Many support groups have a "facilitator," or a professional such as a counselor, nurse, or social worker, who has experience in managing support groups. Successful support groups are supportive—they make the participants feel involved and accepted, regardless of their education, abilities, or personality.

90. What records do I need to keep about my treatment? What is the best way to stay organized?

Although each of your doctors has a record of your treatment, keeping track of what has happened over the course of your treatment is helpful to you, especially if you change doctors or treatment facilities. Some patients write everything in a calendar or notebook. The challenge is to have enough room to write everything that is necessary, and organize it well enough to find information that you may need later. For this reason, many people have found it convenient to use a loose-leaf notebook with dividers to stay

Although each of your doctors has a record of your treatment, keeping track of what has happened over the course of your treatment is helpful to you, especially if you change doctors or treatment facilities.

organized. You may want to keep separate sections for pathology reports, laboratory reports, scan reports, notes from clinic visits, and insurance correspondence. Your doctors will usually be happy to give you copies of your lab and scan reports at your clinic visits. Many imaging facilities now copy magnetic resonance imaging (MRI) or computed tomography (CT) scans on to compact discs; these are very convenient to take to clinic appointments or to mail to consulting physicians. Also, it is useful to keep a one-page summary in your wallet with your current medications, drug allergies, and the names and phone numbers of your doctors. Make sure that the summary includes the dates of your operations and radiation therapy, as well as a list of all of the chemotherapy drugs that you have received. This can be extremely helpful if you have to go to an emergency room when you are away from home.

Many pharmaceutical companies have educational materials including treatment calendars on their websites. The manufacturer of Temodar has also developed a calendar available for Temodar patients that includes stickers to mark doses taken, appointments, scans, and lab tests. In general, any therapy that requires multiple drugs or multiple days of therapy per cycle requires a calendar—as anyone who has ever taken the regimen PCV can attest! If your doctor makes a treatment schedule of your chemotherapy, follow up appointments and scans, ask your doctor if you can have a copy to keep with your records.

M.L.'s comment:

I've met a number of people who had impressive record-keeping systems, including bulky binders with color-coded tabs and graphs of everything from white counts to bowel movements! I can certainly see why so much detail is neces-sary for some patients. Some people may be having a lot of side effects. By keeping careful records of all of the variables involved in their treatment, patients can try to determine what they can change in their treatment to help avoid such toxicity. Also, detailed records are required for clinical trial participants, and patients can expect to be asked about nausea, pain, fatigue, and a number of other side effects that can be difficult to quantitate without careful records.

Initially, keeping track of all of the medications that I was on was quite a challenge. I found it helpful to keep a list of all of my medication, how often I was to take it, and when I was supposed to take it. This was especially important when I was on chemotherapy because I had to take certain medications in a particular order at a particular time. In addition to listing all of my medications, I also listed the day and date so that I could check off when I took my med-ications for that day. When you're taking as many as 10 to 15 pills per day, this type of timetable can be valuable. By keeping this record, I was assured that I wouldn't miss any of my medications.

It was very helpful to take my daily planner with me to every appointment. This was great because it had my cal-endar already in it, along with important names and addresses and extra paper for me to write on. My daily planner also gave me easy access to a list of important ques-tions that I wanted to ask my doctor, and I could write down the answers that my doctors gave me during my visit. For moral support, my husband always went with me to my appointments. If there was something that I missed, he would always remember what was said to me.

I also created a list of my doctors, their telephone numbers, and the names of their nurses or assistants. This became extremely useful when I was receiving radiation treat-ments because I came in contact with at least six other peo-ple in that office (not including my radiation oncologist!). Having my calendar available during radiation treatment helped me to keep track of how many weeks I had been receiving radiation therapy and the appointments that I had for MRI scans. I was able to keep track of the dates of when I would be taking chemotherapy. I'd also be able to make a note to remind myself to have my blood taken the week before chemotherapy so that my oncologist could review the results before I started taking any of the drugs.

Having all of this information available right in my cal-endar made it so much easier for me to communicate infor-mation to my doctors. I found that many times the neurosurgeon, radiologist, and oncologist asked me the same questions. Being able to flip to my calendar without hav-ing to remember all of the information off the top of my head was invaluable to me.

91. My oncologist told me that even though I'm doing well, my tumor will probably come back at some point. He said, "Hope for the best, but prepare for the worst." I'm hoping for the best, but how do I prepare for the worst?

There are many ways that you can mentally and physi-cally prepare yourself for the possible recurrence of your tumor. Follow up with your doctor regularly for physical examinations and possible re-evaluation by MRI or other tests. If your tumor recurs and it can be surgically resected, you should not assume that the sec-ond operation will be identical to the first. Some patients heal more slowly after radiation therapy, but some recover sooner because the recurrent tumor may be smaller than the original. In some cases, the tumor may change to a different subtype more aggressive than the original tumor. This may require additional treatment after surgery.

If your tumor recurs and cannot be removed, your doctor may refer you to a clinical trial or offer you treatment with radiation therapy or chemotherapy if you have not already had these treatments.

Patients with a long interval between their original tumor and a recurrent tumor may be surprised to find that a new treatment is available that had not been available previously; therefore, it is important to discuss with your doctor *at the time of recurrence* how you should be treated. Be prepared, however, to seek a second opinion if your doctor discourages you from pursuing further treatment. Recurrence is not necessarily a death sentence!

It is a fact that some tumors will recur, that further treatments will prove unsuccessful, and that progressive disability will eventually occur. It is also sobering to consider that you may lose the ability to speak or comprehend speech, but some patients do; therefore, you must find someone who will make decisions on your behalf and speak for you. A **Durable Power of Attorney** (DPA) **for Medical Care** allows you to appoint a person who will assume medical decision making for you if you become disabled. Your DPA should have a thorough understanding of your tumor, your prognosis, and your wishes for further treatment if you become incapacitated. Remember that your doctor must be able to contact your DPA if you become incapacitated; it is a good idea to give a copy of your DPA document to your doctor with his or her current phone numbers.

Taking Control of Your Future

Durable Power of Attorney (DPA) for Medical Care
A legal document that allows a specific family member or other adult to legally make decisions for medical care if the patient becomes incapacitated.

A Durable Power of Attorney (DPA) for Medical Care allows you to appoint a person who will assume medical decision making for you if you become disabled.

Another "worst-case scenario" that you should consider is the possibility of sudden incapacity that requires life support. Sometimes complications, such as pulmonary embolus, stroke, and seizures, require temporary support from ventilators, cardiac resuscitation, and intravenous nutrition. If you do not want to receive life support indefinitely, tell your DPA. You may want to develop an **advance directive**, a legal document that specifies whether you want specific kinds of supportive care and for how long. Most hospitals now ask patients on admission if they have a DPA for medical care and an advance directive.

Advance directives

Legal documents that state an individual's preferences for selecting the aggressiveness of supportive care in case of a life-threatening illness.

Understandably, many patients do not want to appoint a DPA or complete an advance directive, reasoning that these tasks should be put off until they are "necessary"; however, it is important to consider these decisions when you are not physically or emotionally stressed. It is particularly important to discuss your concerns with your doctor, as he or she will be able to help you understand what physical limitations you may experience.

For example, one brain tumor patient stated in his advance directive that he did not want any form of "life support." When hospitalized with a severe infection, his blood pressure became dangerously low, although he was still awake and alert. "We could give you medication to keep your blood pressure up," his doctor stated, "but that would mean transferring you to the intensive care unit (ICU) and giving you medication to keep your blood pressure up." The patient was baffled. "Then why don't you do that?" "You said in your advance directive that you didn't want artificial means to keep you alive, and those drugs are considered life support," the doctor answered. "I didn't really mean it! Don't let me die!" the man cried. Fortunately, the patient responded well to the therapy but this case illustrates the potential pitfalls of trying to predict the outcome of severe illness. If the man had been in a coma, dying of his brain tumor, allowing him to die without further intervention may have been the most humane choice.

Another controversy that has become more common in recent years is the role of supplemental nutrition, either with a tube inserted into the stomach, or with intravenous feeding, known as total parenteral nutrition (TPN). Because swallowing can be permanently impaired without affecting consciousness, it is possible that a patient will need "artificial" feeding for the remainder of his or her life. Well-publicized cases of severely brain-injured patients who are kept alive for months or years with "artificial" nutrition should not be confused with the much more common situation of the patient who cannot coordinate swallowing because of dysfunction of the tongue, throat muscles, and nerves. Patients who attempt swallowing despite their doctor's recommendation risk choking and aspiration pneumonia. Even in the case of a dying patient, administering medication such as pain medication, seizure medication, or sedatives may be necessary, and the insertion of a feeding tube may be the easiest and least expensive way to administer such medication in the home or hospice setting. Typically, intravenous nutrition is reserved for patients who have severe gastrointestinal problems and cannot tolerate liquid nutrition through a feeding tube. Total parenteral nutrition is far more expensive and more difficult to maintain than liquid feeding and medications given with a stomach tube.

Occasionally, the terminology used by professionals in discussing a patient's prognosis is less precise than it should be, leading to confusion and even despair.

For example, one brain tumor patient was told immediately after diagnosis by his neurosurgeon that he
needed to "put his affairs in order" because he was "terminal." "I thought you said you took out all of the tumor
and that I need radiation therapy and chemotherapy," he
responded. "You do," replied the neurosurgeon. "Despite
that, you're still going to die. You're terminal." The
patient mentioned the conversation to his radiation
oncologist. "Actually, that's not exactly accurate," the
oncologist answered. "By 'terminal' he probably meant
'incurable,' and you are neither. Even the most aggressive
brain tumors can sometimes be cured, and no one knows
whether you will be cured. Your neurosurgeon obviously
believes that your illness is very serious, and he wanted to
impress on you that it can be fatal; however, 'terminal'
when applied to a patient, means that without life support, the patient will die." "So, I'm not terminal?" the
patient asked. "Not anymore than I am," came the reply.

These cases are illustrative of the common misunder-
standings of patients and their physicians and the limitations of "boilerplate" wording in advance directives. To
"hope for the best and prepare for the worst," patients
must carefully communicate their desires to their DPAs
and physicians so that all parties understand—even if
they do not agree with—the patient's wishes.

92. I did not have a neuropsychological evaluation before surgery, but my neurologist recommended that I have one now that I have completed radiation therapy. How can neuropsychological tests help me?

M.L.'s comment:

*After my surgery, my neurologist suggested that I see a neu-
ropsychologist for testing in order to find out whether my*

surgery caused any temporary or permanent neurological damage. This evaluation process lasted all day. The tests that were performed went beyond the basic testing that was done when my brain tumor was first discovered. The neuropsychological evaluation primarily consisted of a series of paper-and-pencil, question-and-answer tests that are designed to examine various aspects of how the brain functions. My neurologist felt that this type of testing was critical in determining whether I would have problems performing common tasks such as balancing my checkbook. The tests would also determine how my short- and long-term memory had been affected by the surgery, if I would be able to return to work, what limitations I might have, and how I would be able to address those limitations.

Some of the tests were very challenging and frustrating at times, but they varied in content and were not scored on a pass/fail basis; therefore, I knew that it was important for me to put forth my best effort on all of the tests.

I was pleasantly surprised when I got the results back. I was expecting the worst, but the results indicated that my memory (verbal and recall) was very good. I was ranked in the 95th percentile! My attention span and capacity had also remained very strong, but the neuropsychologist strongly recommended that I not push myself too hard because fatigue could affect my attention span. This turned out to be true. When I don't take frequent breaks from the computer or when it's late in the afternoon and I've had a fairly busy day with a lot of meetings, my planning and organization skills "slow down" a bit. I'll end up filing something in the wrong folder or I will forget where I put an important document. Because I'm aware of this potential problem, I try to make sure that I do take frequent breaks from my computer. I also try not to schedule intense or long meetings after about 2 p.m.

Taking Control of Your Future

I have had a few occasional challenges in the area of "language skills." In general, the test results indicated that my language skills were very good to excellent; however, because my tumor was in my left frontal lobe, the area of the brain where language and memory functions are located, there are times when I search for a particular word and I just can't find it. The neuropsychologist warned me that I might encounter this problem; however, the impact has been minimal. I just get a little frustrated at times. I'm usually the only one who really notices it anyway!

Initially, I wasn't looking forward to the neuropsychological tests (for obvious reasons), but when I look back I'm so glad that I took them. The results have given me so much insight in terms of what to expect with my recovery. If I hadn't taken the tests, I wouldn't have known what problems to expect and, more importantly, how to deal with them. The neuropsychologist was excellent in preparing me for my return to a normal life. I learned that when issues do come up I shouldn't panic or let my emotions get the best of me. I would strongly recommend a neuropsychological evaluation for all brain tumor patients.

93. How do I discuss prognosis with my doctor?

Prognosis is the expectation of survival related to the presence of a disease.

Prognosis is the expectation of survival related to the presence of a disease. Your doctor relies on knowledge obtained from the medical literature and personal experience to guide a patient and family through treatment. Doctors are typically reluctant to discuss prognosis until several facts are known: the exact type of tumor, how much of it can be surgically removed, and whether any complications or conditions might affect treatment. The age of the patient and the overall health of the patient also affect the prognosis.

If you are a newly diagnosed patient, you are probably unfamiliar with many terms, such as remission, partial remission, response, stable disease, disease progression, and progression-free survival. Doctors use these to describe the objective evidence of the tumor and to describe the length of time before the tumor recurs. Doctors do not use these terms to avoid discussing a cure; they use such terms to define more accurately the probability that the tumor is present, even when it may not cause symptoms or appear on scans.

Patients often want to know if they can be cured. The answer to that question is never "no," but it may be "it is unlikely." Even in patients with slow-growing brain tumors, the goal of treatment may be to control the symptoms and prevent neurological disability rather than cure the disease.

"Cure" is elusive because it is difficult to prove that a tumor will never reappear, even after years of remission. Some tumors appear to be stable for months or years, only to later grow rapidly into a large mass. For this reason, even obtaining scans at regular intervals does not guarantee that a recurrence will be found while the tumor is still very small. The goal of regular imaging is to detect a recurrent tumor *before* the patient has neurological symptoms or permanent disability and possibly intervene before the patient develops symptoms.

Some patients and their families have been told at the time of diagnosis, "He has 2 years" or, perhaps, "weeks to months." Not surprisingly, a patient's reaction may be disbelief, anger, grief, or fear. Some patients immediately seek a second opinion, hoping to hear a better prognosis. In some cases, this is probably a good idea.

The first doctor may have been right, but the timing (e.g., immediately after surgery) may have made it difficult for the patient and family to understand and accept the gravity of the situation. A second opinion may help patients to accept the situation.

If your doctor informs you that you have a tumor associated with a good prognosis *with treatment*, the prognosis is given with the expectation that you will pursue therapy. For example, patients with primary central nervous system (CNS) lymphoma can achieve complete remission that can be sustained for years, but the disease is rapidly fatal without treatment.

Your doctor may be reluctant to give you an exact time frame for life expectancy. The type of tumor, its rate of growth, its response to therapy, and the presence or absence of other medical problems may all impact survival. If a doctor gives a range of weeks, months, or years, this range is based on the expected behavior of the tumor, not the possible complications that may occur.

M.L.'s comment:

Two of the most important things that I learned were (1) DON'T be intimidated by your doctors, and (2) ask questions. I have found that most patients and caregivers have many questions and concerns, and they need to get answers to all of them. Your doctors and nurses are the people you should look to for answers.

Don't expect your doctors to agree, however! In talking with other patients, I've learned that their neurosurgeons were often the least optimistic in predicting prognosis and their oncologists the most optimistic. The reason for this difference, I think, is that many of the newest advances in the treatment of brain tumors come from drugs, vaccines, and other therapies administered by oncologists.

Although the Internet is an incredible resource for information, keep in mind it may not provide answers to some of your specific questions. Every brain tumor is different. Treatment can be different for each patient. I encourage you to ask your doctors and nurses questions that are specific to you and your situation.

My husband and I had so many questions. Our questions were very specific to the tumor type, at first. Then we wanted to know what (if any) additional treatment would be needed after surgery. We had questions about radiation therapy, chemotherapy, other medications, and all of the associated topics within each of those areas. We weren't afraid to ask questions, so we asked every question we had. We felt like we deserved to know the answers. Sometimes I would become frustrated when we would go to a doctor's appointment because my husband would ask so many questions that I couldn't get an opportunity to ask mine. There were a few times when I said, "Hey, do you think you two could be quiet for a minute while I ask a few questions?" Of course, I said it in a joking way.

I learned at the outset that my tumor could return, regardless of my treatment; however, I knew that I wanted to do everything possible to prevent a recurrence. That led me to pursue several more months of treatment, after completing a year of Temodar. At the time I was diagnosed, Temodar was still a fairly new drug, and no one knew whether there was a higher cure rate in patients who received Temodar for 6 months, 12 months, 18 months, or longer. I was tolerating Temodar very well, and for me, I knew that there was a chance that if my tumor recurred, it could involve the speech area, as my tumor was on the left. So, at the time, I made the decision to continue Temodar a little longer, hoping that this would keep me in remission longer. So far, the strategy has worked—I've been in remission for over 9 years!

94. My doctor told me I have a year to live, but I feel fine now. What will happen to me during the next year? How will I die?

Although it may be too much to assume that your doctor is correct, for the purpose of this discussion, we will assume that he based his opinion on knowing the type of tumor you have and its expected response to treatment. Keep in mind that your tumor could respond much better to treatment or much worse than he anticipates, and therefore, his estimate of 12 months may be little more than an educated guess.

Some patients have very large tumors or multiple tumors at the time of diagnosis. If the tumor cannot be surgically removed safely, the remaining tumor must be successfully treated with another form of therapy if the patient is to survive. Radiation therapy may or may not stop the growth of the tumor. Another form of therapy, such as chemotherapy, may sometimes succeed where radiation failed; however, if the tumor continues to grow through all attempts at treatment, it will ultimately prove fatal. Patients who have metastatic tumors to the brain may have many other sites of disease throughout other vital organs; these patients may have more severe complications related to the total "tumor burden." **Tumor burden** refers to the presence of disease distributed throughout the body that literally affects the health of the entire body.

Tumor burden
Presence of disease affecting the health of the entire body.

Patients who have successful surgery to remove the majority of a brain tumor may still have regrowth of the tumor. This may occur locally (in the same area of the brain as the original tumor), or it may spread to another part of the CNS. The ability to control the growth of a new tumor may be limited by the treatment of the original tumor. For example, further radiation may not be possible, or the tumor may have developed resistance to chemotherapy. The symptoms caused by an enlarging tumor may be slowly progressive, such as the gradual onset of weakness and poor coordination. Sometimes patients with enlarging tumors have a more rapid onset of weakness, confusion, or imbalance. In a few instances, the sudden change may be related to bleeding within the tumor. Some unusual types of tumor progression (such as spread within the spinal fluid or the diffuse spread of tumor throughout the brain, a condition referred to as **gliomatosis cerebri**) are so difficult to treat that patients rarely live more than a year.

Patients with all types of cancer may become more vulnerable to complications such as infection, blood clots, and malnutrition. In addition, patients with primary or metastatic brain tumors may suffer seizures, headaches, vomiting, and difficulty swallowing. These conditions may bring on new problems that result in even further disability. A patient who has difficulty swallowing, for example, may choke on food or fluids, which can lead to pneumonia. Pneumonia may cause shortness of breath, fever, and loss of appetite. A patient who feels short of breath is unlikely to have enough energy to keep physically active, but the lack of activity may increase the risk of blood clots in the vessels of the legs. Swelling and pain in the legs may also limit physical activity, confining the patient to bed. Unfortunately,

Taking Control of Your Future

Gliomatosis cerebri
Infiltrative glial tumor involving multiple lobes of the brain.

Patients with all types of cancer may become more vulnerable to complications such as infection, blood clots, and malnutrition.

these complications may require frequent hospital or emergency room visits. It may be difficult to anticipate and prevent these complications or to reverse many of these conditions once they occur. It is estimated that 70% of cancer patients die of complications, such as infection, rather than the cancer directly.

No one likes to think about such complications when feeling well, but it is helpful nonetheless to talk frankly with one's doctor about the possibility of becoming progressively disabled. The patient and doctor can agree on a hospital that will be used, if necessary, and a nursing service that can provide care at home. It is also important to discuss with family members the aggressiveness of supportive care desired. Advance directives (see Question 91) are instructions to doctors and caregivers specifying whether life-support equipment, artificial nutrition, and other supportive measures should be used if you become too disabled to further direct your care.

It is often difficult to discuss the possibility of deterioration and death with a spouse, a parent, or other family members. One brain tumor patient found that his wife would change the subject every time he mentioned writing an advance directive or learning about hospice care. He was careful to write down his concerns and preferences in a notebook, and matter-of-factly discussed why he did not want to be on life-support equipment. He stated that he did not want any measures such as artificial feeding if he was incapable of regaining consciousness. He investigated inpatient hospices covered by his insurance, as well as the advantages and disadvantages of home hospice. Finally, he gave examples of patients he had heard or read about who had peaceful deaths because their families honored their wishes. He encouraged his wife to read his notebook and even add comments and concerns of her own. In this way, an emotionally charged discussion could take place over days and weeks, with fewer tears on both sides.

95. My neurosurgeon, radiation oncologist, neurologist, and medical oncologist don't always agree. Who is in charge?

The answer might surprise you: You are in charge. Although your doctors may have several years of experience in their respective specialties, it is still up to you to weigh their recommendations. If your doctors are giving you conflicting answers, make sure you find out why.

A common area of disagreement among doctors regards the frequency of follow-up MRI scans. Your neurosurgeon may suggest that you have scans done at 3-month intervals. Your oncologist, on the other hand, may recommend that you have scans done after a specific number of cycles of chemotherapy. Some drugs, such as BCNU and CCNU, are given every 6 to 8 weeks. Other drugs, such as Temodar, are given in 4-week cycles. Your oncologist may change the time between scans to coincide with your chemotherapy cycles. Keep in mind that your doctors may differ in their recommendations for appropriate follow-up, and thus, you may need to remind one doctor of the follow-up procedures that your other doctor has already scheduled. For example, if you do not remind your radiation oncologist that your neurologist has already ordered an MRI, you could be scheduled for MRIs on different days at different facilities!

Another area of vital importance is your medication profile. Although all of your doctors want and need a current medication profile, it is up to you to know exactly which medications you are taking. You are also responsible for making sure that you have enough refills. If you are taking anticonvulsant medication, your neurologist may ask for blood tests to check the level of the drug. If you are also taking chemotherapy, you may be able to arrange for these blood tests to be done when the laboratory tests prescribed by your oncologist are done. If you make sure all of your doctors are aware of the laboratory tests you need, you might be able to save yourself some time—and a needle stick, too.

Some specialists keep their colleagues informed of a patient's progress through letters and phone calls. Others depend on the patient to relay information to the other doctors involved in his or her care. If you find that one of your doctors seems to be unaware of recommendations that another doctor has made, bring this to the doctor's attention immediately. It may be a simple matter of a delay in the transcription and mailing of dictated letters or notes. By keeping copies of your scan reports and laboratory tests, you can update any of your doctors who are temporarily "out of the loop."

M.L.'s comment:

In my situation, I decided that my neuro-oncologist should direct my follow-up. The reason for this was knowing that recurrence was a possibility. Although I have not experienced a recurrence, I do know that tumors can grow very fast (e.g., double or triple in size in a matter of weeks). If my oncologist tells me to get another MRI scan or a PET [positron emission tomography] scan because of an unusual spot that showed up on my last MRI scan . . . then I'm am going to follow up on her advice as soon as possible.

96. My doctor told me that my treatment is not working and that I should consider hospice. If I choose hospice, isn't that just giving up?

Hospice services vary in different communities, but in general, hospice allows patients to receive care for the symptoms of their disease when treatment options to cure or control the disease are unavailable or no longer effective. For example, a woman who has a recurrent brain tumor has undergone surgery, radiation therapy, and chemotherapy. During her last chemotherapy cycle, she had frequent complications requiring hospitalization. This particular patient may not benefit from additional therapy because her quality of life has been compromised by complications. If there are no further treatment alternatives that are likely to be of benefit or if all treatment options appear to be equally toxic, she may be offered hospice.

A physician referral is necessary for patients to be admitted to hospice because patients must meet certain criteria to be eligible. Some of the criteria include life expectancy of 6 months or less, the patient and family are no longer seeking curative measures (only palliative care), and a **DNR** order from the physician.

Hospice services provide care for patients in the home; however, it is important to understand that hospices typically train family members or others within the home to continue to be the primary caregiver. Hospice personnel may visit once or twice a week, increasing the frequency of visits as the patient's condition requires. Hospice nurses work closely with doctors so that symptoms such as seizures, headaches, fever, shortness of breath, and pain are controlled with medications or

DNR

Do not resuscitate. A physician's order to forego life support procedures in the event of cardiac or respiratory arrest. Also called "No Code Blue" or "Allow Natural Death".

other interventions. Hospice services may be paid for by government programs or by private insurance. Some communities have hospice services available for indigent patients.

Do not think of hospice services as giving up an opportunity for effective treatment. In fact, before entering hospice, a patient must be completely sure and comfortable that nothing else can be done to treat his or her tumor. Doctors typically do not refer their patients to hospice care if further treatment is likely to succeed. Acceptance of this prognosis is an important requirement for patients entering hospice.

Hospices commonly have social workers, counselors, and chaplains available to help patients discuss financial concerns and end-of-life decisions. Patients and hospice workers often develop close friendships because of their frequent contact. This relationship can be a great comfort to many patients. Hospice workers also work with surviving family members after the death of the patient to help them cope with the loss.

Hospice workers are trained to alleviate symptoms. They do not do anything to hasten death; however, the use of intravenous fluids, intravenous antibiotics, and artificial feedings are generally discouraged in terminally ill patients because these measures do not ease suffering.

Because patients on hospice do not receive diagnostic testing or expensive treatments, home hospice is far less expensive than hospitalization and continued treatment. Some patients may feel pressured to accept hospice for this reason. Also, in many communities, multiple hospice organizations are available, and competition for patient referrals may be fierce. This may lead to aggressive marketing tactics and a tendency to sign up patients whose needs cannot be met by hospice. For example, many brain tumor patients require anticonvulsants as the tumor progresses, and if the patient is unable to swallow, these medications may have to be given intravenously or by suppository. For this reason, insertion of a feeding tube may be necessary to facilitate "end-of-life" care. Unfortunately, all too often, hospices do not have the appropriate medications or enough experienced personnel to manage them. Although most hospices manage pain effectively, the unique medical needs of a patient must be carefully addressed before the hospice consents are signed. A tragic example of seizure management in an ill-prepared hospice is found in the biography *Same Kind of Different as Me*. With some foresight and planning, almost all patients can be successfully managed in the home situation; however, some patients must be managed in the inpatient setting because the medical problems that they experience are too complicated in the outpatient setting. Status epilepticus, severe uncontrolled pain, or unexpected bleeding may require admission to a hospital or, if available, an inpatient hospice. An inpatient hospice may be a freestanding facility or be a dedicated wing of a hospital. While many communities now have inpatient hospice facilities, some facilities have limited space and are limited to very brief stays.

How does one select a hospice? In some communities, only one hospice is available; however, in larger communities, many hospices may be available. Make sure that the hospice is contracted with the patient's insurance or health plan. Whenever possible, obtaining a recommendation from a friend, support group member or facilitator, or physician who may have had personal experience with a hospice should always be the first step. In fact, if

For example, many brain tumor patients require anticonvulsants as the tumor progresses, and if the patient is unable to swallow, these medications may have to be given intravenously or by suppository.

Taking Control of Your Future

you are anticipating that hospice may be necessary at some point, researching your choices in advance can avoid some of the pitfalls of making a decision too hastily. Interview several hospice representatives, if possible, before making your final choice. Avoid making a decision during the initial interview until you have carefully read all of the documents that you will sign. After you have selected a hospice, if it is not providing the care you need, it may be necessary and perfectly acceptable to change hospices. Hospice care should be compassionate, competent, and readily available to support you and your loved ones.

M.L.'s comment:

Determining whether hospice is the right next step is different for everyone, as there are many things to consider (e.g., the age of the patient, their previous treatment complications, and overall health). The patient and family need to be sure that no other treatment options are desired. You must ask yourself, "Is this the right thing to do for me, or am I doing this because I don't want to be a burden to my family and friends?" If hospice is the right thing to do, the caregiver needs to understand that his or her responsibilities will not decrease. In fact, they will more than likely increase as the patient's ability to care for himself or herself begins to decrease. This is another reason that the caregiver role is so important. Table 10 provides guidelines to assist the patient and the caregiver when selecting a hospice.

Other hospice services could be under the name of Crisis Care, Critical Care, Continual Care, 11th Hour Care, and typically, this service provides round-the-clock care when the patient reaches the point of impending death. This type of support can be critical for a family as they typically are not emotionally equipped

Table 10   Questions to Ask before Entering Hospice

Who is your medical director and what are his/her qualifications?

Will my doctor be consulted regarding my care, or will I be under the care of the hospice doctor?

How many times per week will a nurse visit the home? How many times will another caregiver be available?

Will assistance be available for bathing, feeding, changing linens, etc.? How frequent will this be offered?

Do you have a 24-hour pharmacy available? How long does it take to get a medication after it has been ordered?

How will medications be given if the patient cannot swallow?

Who decides which medications should be administered?

Is there inpatient or respite care available, if the patient's primary caregiver can no longer care for the patient?

Are other services are available (especially with a *for profit* hospice)?

to provide the needed care at such a difficult time. Be aware that many nonprofits do not have the budget to provide this type of service. Twenty-four/seven care is very expensive and demanding, and most hospices do not offer this level of support for more than a few days. In rare cases, the patient may even have to be hospitalized if pain, seizures, or other severe symptoms cannot be controlled despite continuous care in the home.

Some hospices include volunteer programs to stay with the patient while the caregiver does grocery shopping, letter writing, or takes a much needed break from being the sole caregiver. Be sure to ask about "respite care" offered by the hospice, which may allow the patient to be cared for in an inpatient hospice unit while the primary caregiver is out of town or ill.

97. I've been in remission for over 2 years and want to do something to help other brain tumor patients. What can I do?

Good question! First, make sure that your physicians know that you are interested in learning what you can do to help other patients. Your physicians may know of a speaking opportunity, support group, or wellness community where you can share your story. If public speaking is not your thing, you can still offer to write for a patient newsletter or offer your phone number or e-mail address to a newly diagnosed patient who might benefit from your emotional support and firsthand experience.

It can be helpful to begin by writing where you have been and what you have learned since your diagnosis. How has having a brain tumor changed your life? How do you view your life now? How has having a brain tumor changed your family? What has been keeping you going through the low times? How has your impression of health care changed? How can you encourage those who have been less fortunate? Ask your friends and family for their input on how you have grown and changed since your diagnosis.

It is a good time to reflect on people who may have helped you through your treatment and to make sure that you thank them for their concern and support. If you needed transportation or help with insurance forms, did you thank the person who took the time to help? Can you now do something to help her? (If you did not need help, remember that most people do; consider whether it would be possible to help another brain tumor patient make it to his appointments.)

One caregiver who lost his wife to a brain tumor despite years of clinical trials and experimental treatments put his expertise to use when his daughter's boyfriend developed a rare malignancy. He was able to help plan treatments and obtain medications that otherwise would have been impossible for the young man. This type of intervention can cause extreme emotional pain, as the caregiver again takes the time to investigate the treatment alternatives; however, the patient is receiving the benefit of his experience, a gift that no amount of money could buy.

Never forget that local and national organizations (and even international organizations, the International Brain Tumor Association) can use your skills. Every organization needs to raise money—some for brain tumor research, some to help noninsured patients pay their bills—and even if you do not have money, you can help with fund-raising by volunteering your time.

Read about other patients and how they were able to reach out to others. Some patients have developed walk-a-thons, golf tournaments, art shows, benefit concerts, and other events to raise money for those less fortunate. The American Brain Tumor Association, the National Brain Tumor Foundation, and many other organizations raise money for research and education; other organizations, such as the Legacy Brain Foundation, raise money for direct support of brain tumor patients who are unable to afford their treatment. Although there are many technical aspects of starting and maintaining a nonprofit organization in your own community, it can be done, and you will likely meet a number of people, like yourself, who have found truth in the adage, "It is more blessed to give than to receive."

Taking Control of Your Future

98. I was told that my tumor is rare, and it has been difficult to find information about it. How can I find out more about my tumor?

Trying to find information about any kind of brain tumor can be a daunting task. The Internet has simplified the process greatly. People who were diagnosed with a brain tumor just 10 or 15 years ago did not have this valuable resource available to them. Internet resources, such as Yahoo and Google, offer easy-to-use search tools that will lead you to numerous web pages that focus specifically on brain tumors. Of course, you can always consult your local library or the medical library at your local hospital or university, but by far the fastest way to find information is via the Internet. Keep in mind that your doctor should be your primary source of information and will likely have additional medical resources through professional websites and search engines.

Internet resources, such as Yahoo and Google, offer easy-to-use search tools that will lead you to numerous web pages that focus specifically on brain tumors.

When researching your tumor, you must know the exact name of it. You can find the tumor name in your pathology report. For example, it is not enough to know that you have a pineal tumor. Your tumor may be a pineocytoma, a pineoblastoma, a germ-cell tumor, or another type. If your pathology report uses a modifier such as "anaplastic," "malignant," or "metastatic," you must include these terms in your search.

If you enter the term "central neurocytoma" into the search engine at www.google.com, the site currently retrieves over 15,000 references. You can refine these search results by adding other key words or phrases, for example, "central neurocytoma patient education." This retrieves more than 750 references; one in particular is www.righthealth.com, which provides everything you need to know about central neurocytoma—basic resources, media, news and blogs, opinion and discussion, top websites, and more.

Finding more detailed information about central neurocytomas is also possible through medical databases such as Medline or Cancerlit, but if you are interested in a broad discussion of the treatment of central neurocytoma (surgical resection, radiation therapy, and long-term prognosis), you should consider limiting your search to review articles. For most medical literature, only a short summary of the article (the **abstract**) is available online, but the entire article can be obtained from a medical library.

Abstract

Brief summary of a scientific paper.

99. What can I expect in the future in terms of brain cancer treatments?

Now, more than ever before, brain tumor patients have every reason to be optimistic about the future. With the approval of Avastin for the treatment of glioblastoma in 2009, another drug was added to the list of approved drugs (the first since Temodar was approved in 1999). Although many drugs are used off-label and it is anticipated that this practice will continue, the approval of drugs is necessary to ensure that patients will have access to medication through private and federal insurance programs.

Many other targeted therapies are on the horizon—some, like Avastin, targeting angiogenesis and others targeting other genes. Also, newer ways of giving drugs, such as convection-enhanced delivery; and immune-based therapies, such as the tumor vaccines, are becoming available at many centers. Some drugs are oral and some are intravenous; some can be added to existing standard treatments.

Also, more hospitals across the country are installing imaging systems such as intraoperative MRIs to allow more complete resection of brain tumors. New agents are also being developed that stain brain tumor cells specifically, allowing the surgeon to see small areas of residual tumor, even without special imaging.

Over the past 5 years, advances in radiation therapy have also become more available. Cyberknife, Gamma Knife, and other highly conformal radiation techniques allow radiation treatments now that would have been more difficult a few years ago. Finally, many other advances, including new anticonvulsants, better diagnostic imaging, and even newly discovered genes, will continue to impact brain tumor treatment for years to come.

Even more astounding, some of these advances were first proposed by brain tumor patients and caregivers. Dr. Ben Williams, a brain tumor survivor who has published extensively on the use of drug cocktails, has continued to encourage the use of multiagent therapies for brain tumors. The first use of Avastin in glioblastoma was actually proposed by a patient and her husband, who had read about the drug's success in colon cancer. The Society of Neuro-Oncology, the U.S. professional association of neurologists, neurosurgeons, neuro-oncologists, radiation oncologists, and other neuroscientists, has recently opened its professional meetings to allow patients to hear the latest research findings presented.

100. Where can I go for further information?

Many hospitals and cancer centers have patient libraries and resource centers with booklets and reading lists about specific topics. In addition, The American Brain Tumor Association (www.abta.org), the American Cancer Society (www.cancer.org), the National Cancer Institute (www.cancer.gov), and National Institutes of Health (www.nih.gov), just to name a few, publish a variety of books about clinical trials, cancer diagnosis and treatment, and nutritional support for cancer patients. Booklets are available free of charge by calling: 1-800-4CANCER.

The web portal www.virtualtrials.com is one of the most comprehensive brain tumor information sites on the web. This incredible resource lists clinical trials, results of studies, and many articles of interest to the brain tumor patient and caregiver. The weekly "Brain Tumor News Blast" is offered to subscribers from virtualtrials.com and presents current information about drugs under development, fund-raising events for brain tumor patients, and other news.

Also, a number of excellent books have been published over the last several years. See the Appendix for an updated list of books and references.

Booklets are available free of charge by calling: 1–800–4CANCER.

Taking Control of Your Future

National Organizations for Brain Tumor Patients

American Brain Tumor Association
2720 River Road, Suite 146
Des Plaines, IL 60018
Phone: 847-827-9910
www.abta.org
Provides information free of charge about brain tumors and sponsors research grants and regional "Town Hall Meetings." The gray ribbon "Brain Tumor Awareness" lapel pin is available from the ABTA store.

The National Brain Tumor Society
124 Watertown Street, Suite 3H
Watertown, MA 02472-2500
Phone: 800-770-8287
West Coast Office
22 Battery Street, Suite 612
San Francisco, CA 94111-5520
www.braintumor.org
A website that includes information about events and conferences, including teleconferences and live web casts. An extensive book list about brain tumors and brain tumor survivors is available by request and online.

Pediatric Brain Tumor Foundation of the United States
315 Ridgefield Court
Asheville, NC 28806
Phone: 800-253-6530
www.pbtfus.org
Promotes public awareness of pediatric brain tumors and raises money in support of adult and pediatric brain tumor research.

Brain Tumor Foundation for Children, Inc.
6065 Roswell Road, Suite 505
Atlanta, GA 30328-4015
Phone: 404-252-4107
www.braintumorkids.org
A nonprofit organization to promote awareness and support research for children with brain tumors.

Candlelighters Childhood Cancer Foundation
10400 Connecticut Avenue, Suite 205
Kensington, MD 20895
Phone: 800-366-2223
www.candlelighters.org
A resource for families of children with cancer.

Other Useful Resources and Websites

National Center for Complementary and Alternative Medicine
P.O. Box 8218
Silver Spring, MD 20907
Phone: 301-435-5042
www.nccam.nih.gov
This site contains information about complementary and alternative medicine, including current clinical trials using these methods.

American Cancer Society
1599 Clifton Road, NE
Atlanta, GA 30329
Phone: 800-ACS-2345
www.cancer.org
A website that is easy to use and has
  information on a wide variety of topics,
  including chemotherapy and radiation
  therapy.

**Musella Foundation for Brain Tumor
Research and Information**
www.virtualtrials.com
This is a fantastic resource for anyone newly
  diagnosed with a brain tumor, anyone
  starting chemotherapy or radiation therapy, or someone who is looking for a
  clinical trial. It is well-organized and regularly updated and may be the only brain
  tumor resource you will ever need. It also
  has links to many other useful sites.

NeedyMeds
www.needymeds.com
If you cannot afford your medication, this
  site can give you some useful resources,
  sometimes free from the manufacturer.

Oncolink
www.oncolink.com
This site, sponsored by the Abramson
  Cancer Center of the University of
  Pennsylvania, contains information on
  a wide variety of cancer topics, including
  clinical trials.

Vital Options International
www.vitaloptions.org
An international organization for young
  adults with cancer, hosting a weekly
  syndicated radio show and web cast on
  a variety of topics.

CancerCare
www.cancercare.org
CancerCare is a nonprofit organization
  providing free professional help to
  patients with all types of cancers. This
  website includes information for
financial assistance, support groups,
cancer and sexuality, and many other
topics.

CancerSource.com
www.cancersource.com
This is a well-illustrated and comprehensive resource for cancer patients and
families about diagnosis and treatment
options, including more advanced topics
for nursing and medical professionals.
This site allows you to receive a person-
alized e-mail newsletter. It is partnered
with Jones and Bartlett Publishers,
allowing purchase of books online.

Selected U.S. Cancer Centers with Brain Tumor Programs

Children's National Medical Center
111 Michigan Avenue, NW
Washington, DC 20010
Phone: 202-476-3000
www.cnmc.org

University of Alabama at Birmingham
Birmingham, AL
www.braintumor.uab.edu

**Cedars–Sinai Maxine Dunitz
Neurosurgical Institute**
8700 Beverly Boulevard
Los Angeles, CA 90048
Phone: 310-423-7900
www.cedars-sinai.edu/mdsni

**University of California, Los Angeles
(UCLA) Medical Center**
Los Angeles, CA
Phone: 310-825-5074
www.neurooncology.ucla.edu

University of Southern California
1520 San Pablo Street., Suite 3800
Los Angeles, CA 90089
Phone: 323-442-5720
www.usc.edu/medicine/neurosurgery

University of California at San Francisco
San Francisco, CA
Phone: 415-353-2966
www.ucsf.edu.nabtc.org

**University of Colorado Health
Sciences Center**
Aurora, CO
Phone: 720-848-0116
www.uch.uchs.edu/uccc/patient/neuroonc.html

**H. Lee Moffitt Cancer Center
and Research Institute**
Tampa, FL
Phone: 813-632-1730
www.moffitt.usf.efu/clinical/nonc/index.htm

Brigham & Women's Hospital
Boston, MA
Phone: 617-732-6810
www.boston-neurosurg.org

Massachusetts General Hospital
Boston, MA
Phone: 617-726-7851
www.brain.mgh.harvard.edu

Johns Hopkins Hospital
Baltimore, MD
Phone: 410-955-0703
www.nabtt.org/johns.html

National Cancer Institute
Bethesda, MD
Phone: 301-402-6298
www.dcs.nci.nih.gov/trials

Henry Ford Hospital
Detroit, MI
Phone: 313-916-1340
www.nabtt.org/henry.html

**University of North Carolina–Lineburger
Comprehensive Cancer Center**
Chapel Hill, NC
Phone: 919-966-1374
www.cancer.med.unc.edu

Duke University Medical Center
Durham, NC
Phone: 919-684-5301
www.cancer.duke.edu/btc

Dartmouth–Hitchcock Medical Center
Lebanon, NH
Phone: 603-650-6312
www.dartmouth.edu/dms/nccc/brain.htm

Memorial Sloan–Kettering Cancer Center
New York, NY
Phone: 800-525-2225
www.mskcc.org

New York Presbyterian Hospital
Weill Cornell Medical Center
New York, NY
Phone: 212-746-2438

Children's Hospital of Philadelphia
Philadelphia, PA
Phone: 215-590-3129
www.chop.edu

Children's Hospital of Pittsburgh
Pittsburgh, PA
Phone: 412-692-5881
www.neurosurgery.pitt.edu

St. Jude Children's Research Hospital
Memphis, TN
Phone: 901-495-3604
www.stjude.org/brain

M.D. Anderson Cancer Center
Houston, TX
Phone: 713-794-1285
www.mdanderson.org

**University of Utah/Huntsman
Cancer Institute**
Salt Lake City, UT
Phone: 801-581-6908
www.hci.utah.edu/5065.html

Appendix

University of Wisconsin Medical School
Madison, WI
Phone: 608-263-5009
www.humonc.wisc.edu

Fox Chase Cancer Center
Philadelphia, PA
Phone: 215-717-3005
www.neuro-oncology.org

Other Helpful Organizations

American Institute for Cancer Research
1759 R Street NW
Washington, DC 20009
Phone: 800-843-8114 or 202-328-7744

Americans with Disabilities Act
U.S. Department of Justice
950 Pennsylvania Avenue
Washington, DC 20530
Phone: 800-514-0301
www.usdoj.gov/crt/ada/adahom1.htm

National Coalition for Cancer Survivorship
1010 Wayne Avenue, Suite 505
Silver Spring, MD 20910
Phone: 877-NCCSYES (622-7937)
www.cansearch.org
Acts as a clearinghouse and helps cancer survivors, their families, and friends find local support groups, learn health insurance options, and prevent employment bias.

National Family Caregivers Association
10400 Connecticut Avenue, #500
Kensington, MD 20895
Phone: 800-896-3650
www.nfcacares.org
Provides education, support, respite care, and advocacy for caregivers. Their toll-free information line provides referrals to caregiver support groups as well as information on how to start a caregivers' support group.

National Hospice Organization
Phone: 800-658-8898
www.nho.org
Promotes quality care for the terminally ill and their families. Their help line refers callers to local hospices, and they can also inform callers as to whether a facility is licensed and Medicare-certified.

Patient Advocate Foundation
739 Thimble Shoals Boulevard, Suite 704
Newport News, VA 23606
Phone: 800-532-5274
www.patientadvocate.org

Further Reading

Alive and Fighting: Coping with a Brain Tumor and a Bone Marrow Transplant. H. Charles Wolf. Author House, 2005.
Brain Tumors: Finding the Ark. Paul Zeltzer, MD. Shilysca Press, 2006.
Brain Tumors: Leaving the Garden of Eden. Paul Zeltzer, MD. Shilysca Press, 2004.
Curveball: When Life Throws You a Brain Tumor. Liz Holzemer. Ghost Road Publishing Group, Inc., 2009.
Damn the Statistics, I Have a Life to Live. H. Charles Wolf. Author House, 2003.
Force a Miracle. Darryl C. Didier. iUniverse, 2002.
Living with a Brain Tumor. Peter Black, MD, PhD, FACS. Holt, 2006.
My Fortunate Brain Tumor from God. Dave Jiang. Xulon Press, 2007.
Surviving "Terminal" Cancer. Ben Williams, PhD. Fairview Press, 2002.
Surviving the Cancer System. Mark Fesen, MD, FACP. AMACOM, 2009.

Glossary

Abstract: Brief summary of a scientific paper.

Advance directives: Legal documents that state an individual's preferences for selecting the aggressiveness of supportive care in case of a life-threatening illness.

Alternative therapy: Treatment used in lieu of standard medical therapies.

Anemia: Low red blood cell count; may cause tiredness, weakness, and shortness of breath.

Animal models: Laboratory animals that have diseases similar to those in humans.

Antiangiogenesis: Property of a drug or other treatment that prevents the formation of new blood vessels.

Antiemetic medications: Drugs that prevent nausea and vomiting.

Astrocytes: One of the major types of glial cells of the nervous system.

Astrocytoma: A glioma that has developed from astrocytes.

Axial image: An image that begins at the crown and ends at the base of the skull, revealing the left and right halves of the brain.

Benign: Not cancerous; not life threatening.

Bioavailability: Chemical property of a drug describing its absorption through the gastrointestinal tract when taken orally.

Biopsy: Surgical removal of a small piece of tissue or a tumor for microscopic examination.

Blood–brain barrier: Tightly joined cells in the blood vessels of the brain that prevent the ready diffusion of substances into the brain tissue.

Bone marrow reserve: Term used by oncologists to describe the expectation of recovery of bone marrow cells after treatment with chemotherapy or radiation therapy.

Boost: High dose of fractionated radiation.

Brachytherapy: Internal radiation therapy that involves placing radioactive material near or in the tumor.

Brainstem: That part of the central nervous system responsible for a number of "unconscious" activities, including breathing, heart rate, wakefulness, and sleep.

Broca's area: An area in the frontal lobe of the brain that is associated with speech.

Cancerous: Abnormal and uncontrolled growth of cells in the body that may spread, injure areas of the body, and lead to death.

CentiGray (cGy): Unit of radiation, equal to one rad.

Central nervous system (CNS): Pertaining to the brain and spinal cord.

Cerebellum: Part of the brain located at the back of the head, under the cerebrum, and in back of the brain-stem. Controls balance and coordination, affecting movements of the same side of the body.

Cerebrum: The largest area of the brain; divided into the right and left cerebral hemispheres.

Chemotherapy: The use of chemical agents (drugs) to treat cancer.

Chondrosarcoma: A malignant tumor of the cartilage.

Chordoma: A rare and slow-growing tumor that develops in the spine and base of the skull.

Choroid plexus: Two sponge-like tissues in the lateral ventricles that produce the spinal fluid.

Clinical trial: A research protocol that is designed to answer a question regarding a population of patients with disease or who are at risk for disease.

Cobalt: A radioactive isotope used in the treatment of cancer.

Complementary therapy: Treatment used in conjunction with standard treatment for disease.

Complete remission (CR): Complete resolution of all signs and symptoms of disease.

Computed tomography (CT): Computerized series of X-rays that create a detailed cross-sectional image of the body.

Conformal radiation therapy: Three-dimensional radiation using images from a CT scan and an MRI to plan precise fields of radiation that may be contoured around structures such as the eyes or the brainstem.

Convection enhanced delivery: A treatment technique in which drugs are administered through small catheters directly into the area surrounding a tumor.

Conventional radiation: The type of radiation therapy delivered by a linear accelerator, usually divided over several treatments.

Coronal image: Image that divides the brain into front (anterior) and back (posterior) and shows the best deeper and more central areas of the brain.

Corpus callosum: A prominent nerve fiber bundle in the center of the brain connecting the cerebral hemispheres.

Cortex: The outer surface of the cerebral hemispheres; often called the gray matter.

Corticosteroid: A naturally occurring hormone produced by the adrenal cortex, or a synthetic hormone having similar properties; often used to treat edema (swelling) in leaky capillaries of the brain.

Cranial nerves: Nerves that arise from the base of the brain or the brainstem that provide sensory and motor function to the eyes, nose, ears, tongue, and face.

Craniotomy: A surgical "cutting" of an opening into the skull.

Cyclotron: A circular particle accelerator. Ion beams created with a cyclotron can be used in proton therapy as a cancer treatment.

Deep vein thrombosis (DVT): Blood clot forming in deep veins, often with impaired or sluggish blood flow.

Deoxyribonucleic acid (DNA): The genetic information in the cell nucleus, containing directions on cell growth, division, and function.

DNR: Do not resuscitate. A physician's order to forego life support procedures in the event of cardiac or respiratory arrest. Also called "No Code Blue" or "Allow Natural Death".

Dominant: Ruling or controlling. The cerebral hemisphere that controls speech formation is referred to as the dominant hemisphere.

Durable Power of Attorney (DPA) for Medical Care: A legal document that allows a specific family member or other adult to legally make decisions for medical care if the patient becomes incapacitated.

Edema: Swelling or fluid build-up.

Electroencephalogram (EEG): A recording of the electrical impulses of the brain using electrodes attached to the scalp.

Ependymal: One of the major types of glial cells, which line the surfaces of the ventricles of the brain and the center canal of the spinal cord.

Ependymoma: Tumor that has developed from abnormal ependymal cells.

Exclusion criteria: Characteristics specified in a clinical trial that render the patient ineligible for the study.

External beam radiation: The type of radiation therapy delivered by a linear accelerator.

Fields: The volume of tissue to be treated during radiation therapy.

Fissures: The deep folds that separate each cerebral hemisphere into lobes.

Food and Drug Administration (FDA): A federal institution charged with approving and regulating medications, foodstuff, and other products for human consumption.

Foramen magnum: A large hole at the base of the skull; it serves as the boundary between the brainstem and the spinal cord.

Fraction: Single treatment of radiation.

Frontal lobe: The anterior (toward the face) area in the cerebral hemisphere involved in emotion, thought, reasoning, and behavior.

Functional MRI: A type of MRI that detects the changes in red blood cells and capillaries as they deliver oxygen to "functioning" parts of the brain.

Gadolinium: A silvery-white, malleable rare-earth metal that is often used in intravenous compounds that enhance contrast in MRIs and other imaging.

Gamma Knife: Type of stereotactic radiation designed to deliver radiation from multiple cobalt sources, computer-focused to a small area or multiple small areas.

Generalized seizure: Seizure involving both hemispheres of the brain.

Glial cells: Supportive tissue of the brain; includes astrocytes, oligodendrocytes, and ependymal cells. Unlike neurons, they do not conduct electrical impulses and can reproduce.

Glioma: A tumor originating in the neuroglia of the brain or spinal cord.

Gliomatosis cerebri: The diffuse spread of tumor throughout the brain.

Grade: The degree to which tumor tissue resembles normal tissue under the microscope. Tumors are classified as low grade if they are still very similar to normal cells, high grade if they have a rapid growth rate with distorted or disorganized cells, or intermediate grade if they fall in between low and high grades.

Gray (Gy): Modern unit of radiation dosage.

Gross total resection: Removal of all visible portions of a tumor.

Hemisphere: One of the two halves of the cerebrum or the cerebellum.

High grade: Tumor that has a rapid growth rate; the cells may appear disorganized and distorted.

Inferior vena cava (IVC) filter: A vascular filter that is implanted into the inferior vena cava to prevent blood clots in the bloodstream from reaching the heart.

Informed consent: Process of explaining to the patient all risks and complications of a procedure or treatment before it is done. Informed consents are signed by the patient, a parent of a minor child, or a legal representative.

Intermediate grade: Tumors that have features of aggressiveness and growth characteristics between low- and high-grade tumors.

Interstitial brachytherapy: Radiation therapy that is administered from the inside of the tumor cavity, with a source of radiation therapy such as radioactive iodine or iridium.

Intra-arterial administration: Injection into an artery that supplies blood to the tumor.

Intracavitary administration: The administration of a drug directly into the tumor cavity.

Intrathecal administration: The injection of a drug directly into the spinal fluid.

Intraoperative MRI: An "MRI guidance" system available in operating rooms designed to function with an MRI scanner.

Investigational: Treatments that are experimental or under development in clinical trials, including drugs that were approved for other uses.

Investigators: Physicians or other individuals who are involved with an experimental study or clinical trial.

Ionizing radiation: A form of energy that knocks electrons out of their normal orbits.

Lateral ventricles: The two elongated, curved openings in each cerebral hemisphere connecting with two slit-like openings in the center of the brain.

Leptomeningeal metastases: The spread of cancer cells through the spinal fluid, producing a coating around the brain or spinal cord.

Leptomeningeal spread: The spread of cancer cells through the spinal fluid, producing a coating around the brain or spinal cord.

Limbic system: A group of deep brain structures that are associated with emotions, behavior, learning, and memory.

Linear accelerator: A machine used in radiation therapy that is able to create man-made ionizing radiation in the form of X-rays to penetrate through tissue into a tumor.

Localizing: Symptoms suggesting that a specific area of the nervous system is involved, for example, speech disturbance, weakness of one side of the body, or loss of vision.

Low grade: Tumors that have few cells dividing at any one time, often resembling normal tissue.

Lumbar puncture: Method of obtaining a sampling of spinal fluid from the space between the lumbar vertebrae.

Lymphocytes: Type of white blood cell found in lymphatic tissue such as lymph nodes, spleen, and bone marrow.

Magnetic resonance imaging (MRI): A radiographic study based on the acquisition of anatomical information using resonance from atoms in a strong magnetic field.

Magnetic resonance spectroscopy (MRS): A study similar to conventional MRI that measures chemical compounds within the brain.

Malignant: Cancerous; cells that exhibit rapid, uncontrolled growth.

Malignant transformation: The development of more destructive, invasive, or rapid growth in a previously benign or indolent tumor.

Margin: An area around the edge of a tumor visualized on brain scan, which may include scattered tumor cells.

Medical history: A detailed accounting by the patient that helps a physician to determine the length and severity of an illness as well as previous personal and family health history.

Medical oncologist: A physician who performs comprehensive management of cancer patients throughout all phases of care; specializes in treating cancer with medicine.

Meninges: Membranes covering the brain and spinal cord, consisting of the pia, arachnoid, and dura.

Meningioma: A slow-growing tumor of the meninges.

Metabolism: The normal physical and chemical changes within living tissue.

Metastasis: The spread of cancer from the initial cancer site to other parts of the body through the lymphatic system, the bloodstream, or the spinal fluid.

Metastatic tumors: Cancer that has spread outside of the organ or structure in which it arose to another area of the body.

Mini-Mental Status Examination: A brief verbal and written examination that tests orientation, memory, calculation, language, and figure drawing on a 30-point scale.

Monocytes: Type of white blood cells normally found in the lymph nodes, spleen, bone marrow, and within tissue.

Multifocal: Having more than one point of origin.

Myelin: A fatty material that forms a layer around the axon of a neuron and is essential for proper nervous system function.

Necrosis: The premature, localized death of cells and living tissue.

Neurological deficit: Partial or complete loss of muscle strength, sensation, or other brain functions; may be temporary or permanent.

Neurological examination: Part of the physical examination testing general intellectual function, speech, motor function, memory, sensation, reflexes, and cranial nerve functions.

Neuron: Nerve cell that conducts electrical or chemical signals.

Neuronavigation: Preoperative or intraoperative imaging information that allows the surgeon to view images in the operating room during surgery to localize normal brain structures and tumor.

Neuropathologist: Pathologist specializing in the diagnosis of diseases of the peripheral and central nervous systems.

Neuropsychologist: Professionals who specialize in the effect of brain injury on behavior and cognition. They help identify ways to improve relearning and to compensate for neurological functions that are impaired.

Neuroradiologist: Physician trained to interpret X-rays, CT scans, and other radiological images of the brain.

Neurosurgeon: Surgeon specializing in the diagnosis and treatment of disease of the central and peripheral nervous systems, including the skull, spine, and blood vessels.

Neutropenia: A lower than normal neutrophil count.

Neutrophil: Type of white blood cell.

Noncancerous: Tissue that does not appear to be malignant; may be benign or normal.

Nondiagnostic: A tissue sample that does not contain adequate information for determining the presence or absence of disease.

Nonlocalizing: Symptoms not confined, limited, or contained to a specific area; may be attributed to other illnesses, depression, or stress. Examples include fatigue, lack of concentration, or nausea.

Occipital lobe: Area in the cerebral hemispheres that interpret visual images as well as the meaning of written words.

Occupational therapy: Assists patients in normalizing activities of daily living, such as bathing, brushing teeth, cutting meat, and dressing.

Off-label drug: A drug that is approved by the FDA for one type of treatment but may be prescribed for other conditions.

Oligodendrocytes: One of the major types of glial cells.

Oligodendroglioma: Abnormal oligodendrocytes that grow into a tumor.

Ommaya reservoir: A hollow, slightly dome-shaped device is attached to a catheter that is surgically implanted into the cerebral ventricle. Chemotherapy is administered by injection into the reservoir and catheter.

Open biopsy: Procedure allowing a neurosurgeon to directly visualize the surface of the brain prior to the removal of a piece of a tumor.

Parietal lobe: Area in the cerebral hemispheres that controls sensory and motor information.

Partial remission (PR): Shrinkage or partial disappearance of a tumor, but with evidence that some of the tumor still exists.

Partial resection: Procedure that allows a neurosurgeon to directly visualize the surface of the brain prior to removal of some, but not all, of a tumor.

Partial seizure: Seizure involving only one area or lobe of the brain.

Pathologist: A physician trained to examine and evaluate cells, tissue, and organs for the presence of disease.

Pathology report: Summary of the gross (specimen visible to the naked eye) and microscopic analysis of tissue and/or fluid removed during surgery.

Pharmacokinetics: Study of how the body breaks down a drug after it is administered.

Phase I trial: Study of a small group of patients to determine the effectiveness and the side effects of a new treatment.

Phase II trial: Study of a group of similar patients to determine whether there is a statistical likelihood that a new treatment will be effective against a tumor.

Phase III trial: Compares two or more kinds of treatment in two or more similar groups of patients, with one group of patients receiving the standard, or control, therapy.

Physiatrist: Physician who specializes in physical medicine and rehabilitation and in prescribing the components of a rehabilitation program.

Physical therapy: Therapy aimed at recovery from weakness, loss of coordination, or limited endurance.

Pilot study: Small study designed to test an idea or treatment prior to a larger clinical trial; also called a feasibility study.

Placebo: A medication ("sugar pill") or treatment that has no effect on the body, often used in experimental studies to determine if the experimental medication/treatment has an effect.

Positron emission tomography (PET): A nuclear medicine imaging test that detects differences in metabolism; often used to differentiate between healthy and abnormal tissue.

Precentral gyrus: An area of the brain that contains the primary motor cortex, which controls voluntary muscle movement.

Primary brain tumor: Tumors that develop from mutations of normal cells that originate in the brain, the spinal cord, or the meninges.

Prognosis: The long-term outlook for survival and recovery from a disease based on the patient's current status and the anticipated effect of available treatments.

Proliferation index: A measurement of the growth and division rate of cells obtained from a biopsy specimen, using special stains.

Protocol: A research plan for how a therapy is given and to whom it is given.

Proton beam therapy: A cancer therapy that uses a beam of protons to irradiate a tumor while minimizing damage to surrounding healthy tissue.

Pulmonary embolus: Blood clot that travels through the veins and the heart, eventually occluding one or more pulmonary arteries.

Radiation necrosis: An area of injured normal glial cells and blood vessels that may occur several months after radiation therapy.

Radiation oncologist: A physician who specializes in treating cancer with radiation.

Radiation physicist: A scientist trained to determine the dose and accuracy of radiation therapy equipment.

Radiation therapy: Treatment that uses high-dose X-rays or other high-energy rays to kill cancer cells and shrink tumors.

Radiosensitivity: A tumor's susceptibility to growth inhibition or cell killing by radiation therapy.

Radiosignal: In MRI, the image produced by resonance of hydrogen atoms in a magnetic field during and after a radiofrequency pulse.

Radiosurgery: Type of radiation therapy that focuses energy to a small area of a tumor, usually less than 3 to 4 centimeters in diameter. It does not involve surgery.

Randomized trial: Clinical trial involving at least two subgroups of patients comparing two or more different therapies, with the therapy selected by random assignment rather than by the patient or investigator.

Recreational therapist: Assists patients to engage in leisure activities such as cooking, arts and crafts, and music therapy that can provide a cognitive component to the "work" of physical rehabilitation.

Rehabilitation counselor: Assesses the goals of the patient and his or her return to work and family life.

Remission: Complete or partial disappearance of the signs and symptoms of disease in response to treatment; the period during which disease is under control.

Resectable: Able to be surgically removed.

Resection: Surgical removal of a tumor; see also gross total resection and partial resection.

Sagittal image: An image that divides the brain into left and right hemispheres and is particularly good at showing tumors in the exact center of the brain.

Secondary brain tumors: Cancer that has spread, or metastasized to the brain from another organ, such as the lungs.

Secondary malignancy: Cancer that develops as a result of previous cancer therapy.

Simulation: A practice treatment that allows the radiation team to determine exactly where the radiation treatment will be directed.

Speech therapist: Professionals who evaluate speech production, speech comprehension, and swallowing function.

Spinal tap: See lumbar puncture.

Sponsor: The organization that funds a research study or clinical trial.

Status epilepticus: A condition in which the patient has repeated seizures or a seizure prolonged for at least 30 minutes.

Stereotactic biopsy: Removal of a small piece of the tumor using computer guidance, often with a thin needle placed through a tiny opening in the scalp and skull.

Stereotactic radiation: Type of radiation therapy that focuses energy to a small area of a tumor, usually less than 3 to 4 centimeters in diameter. It may be fractionated over several treatments.

Stereotactic radiosurgery (SRS): A radiation therapy technique using a large number of narrow, precisely aimed, highly focused beams of ionizing radiation. Beams aimed from many directions meet at a specific point. Usually only one treatment at a high dose is planned.

Stereotactic radiotherapy: Type of radiation therapy that focuses the dose to a small area of a tumor, usually less than 3 to 4 centimeters in diameter, fractionated over a few days.

Target volume: The three-dimensional portion of an organ or organs, identified from the patient's scans or X-rays, to receive radiation therapy treatments.

Temporal lobe: Area in the cerebral hemispheres that contain both the auditory and visual pathways and the interpretation of sounds and spoken language for long-term memory.

Third and fourth ventricles: Two spinal fluid-filled spaces in the center of the brain in communication with the lateral ventricles.

Thrombocytopenia: Low platelet count.

Tumor burden: The presence of disease distributed throughout the body that affects the health of the entire body.

Turcot's syndrome: An inherited condition associated with colon polyps and brain tumors.

Whole-brain radiation therapy: Radiation therapy delivered to the entire intracranial contents.

Index

Index